THE AUSTRALIAN
AUTOIMMUNE
PROTOCOL
COOKBOOK

Food Is
Life

NATASHA**HORVATH**

Over 100 authentic, Australian AIP compliant
recipes!
All recipe measurements are in both metric
and imperial.

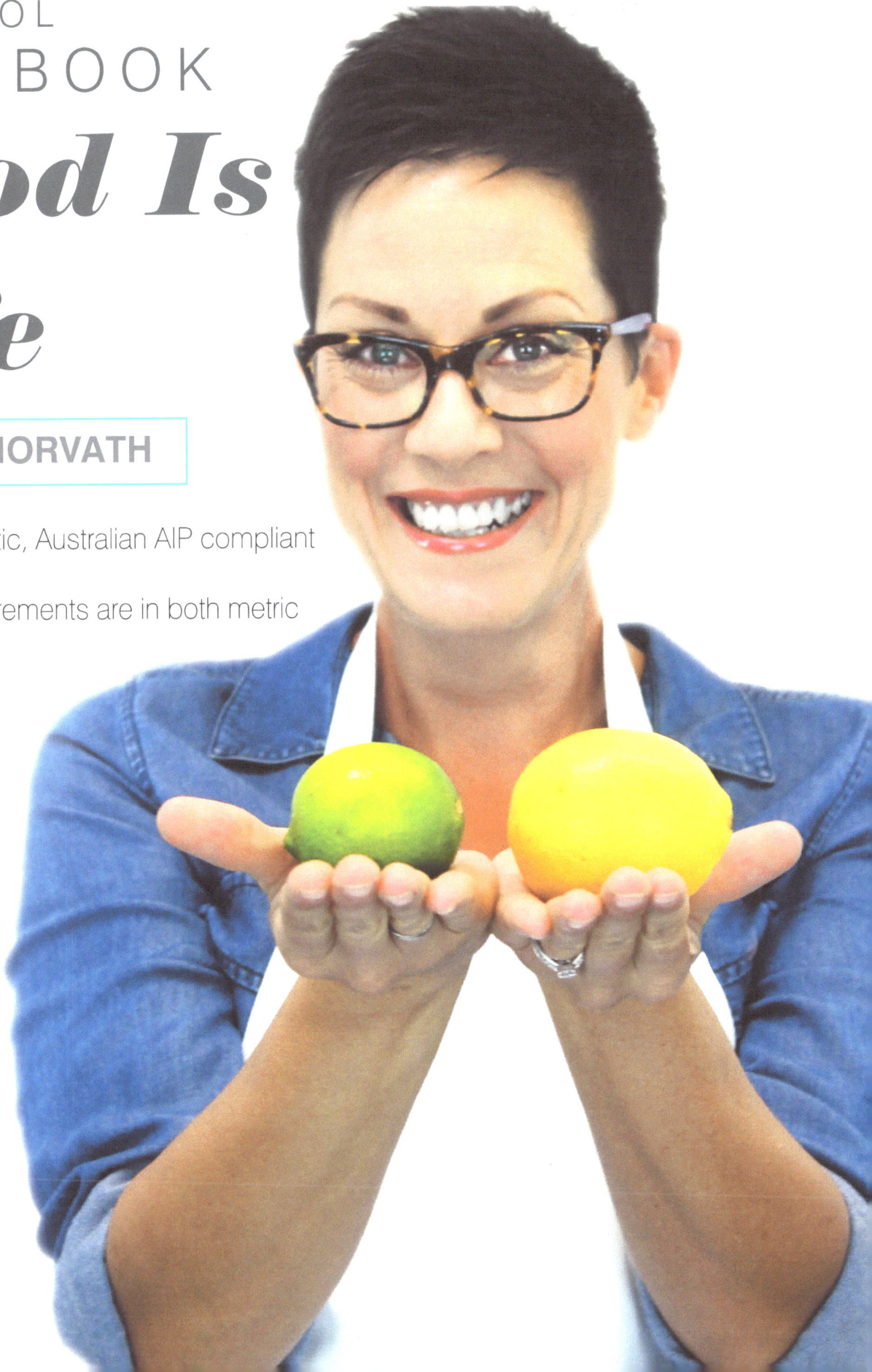

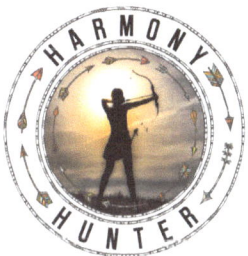

HARMONY
HUNTER

NATASHA**HORVATH**

The Australian Autoimmune Protocol Cookbook

Appreciation

Thank you to all of the AIP champions, who have tirelessly provided information and support for all those affected by autoimmune and chronic illness. The following people have helped me to hunt for my harmony and improve the quality of my life, and have inspired me to write this cookbook.

Thank you to:

Mickey Trescott – www.autoimmune-paleo.com
Dr Sarah Ballantyne – www.thepaleomom.com

Eileen Laird –www.phoenixhelix.com
Dr Terry Wahls –www.terrywahls.com

Disclaimer: The content presented in this book is intended for inspiration and informational purposes only. I am not a Medical Professional and the information contained within this book is not meant to treat, cure, or prevent any disease or illness. Please seek the advice of a qualified Medical Professional before making any dietary changes.

ISBN: 978-0-9945-7979-9 (sc)
ISBN: 978-0-9945-7970-6 (e)

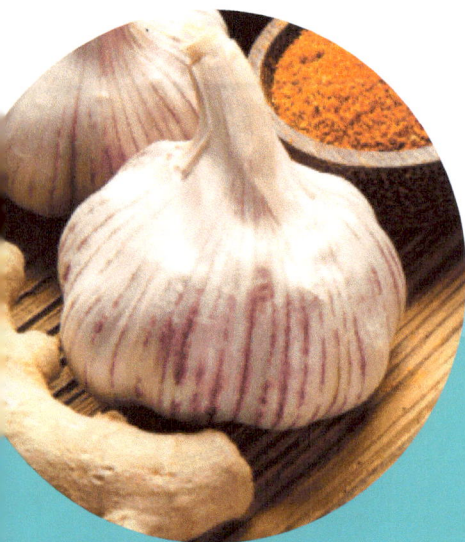

FOREWORD

In the last century we have been witnessing the emergence of a rather new entity of medical conditions called "Autoimmune" disorders, these according to medical books and literature have "unknown etiology" which in a sense has been an ever baffling subject for the profession. Only in the last 15 years the literature has been able to suggest that what breaks our immune barrier mostly penetrates our system from the largest front in our body, the" Gut". Thanks to the work of researchers like Bonnie Basler's group in MIT, the idea of gut microbiome and the effects of bacterial epigenetics on our lives started to gain a lot of momentum.

The recent publication from faecal transplant research has been extremely overwhelming and somewhat unexplainable to the medical profession to the point that gut microbiota is now linked with depression, anxiety, obesity, anorexia, etc., and in a nut shell the research is suggesting it is "the cure of all conditions"!

The advent of faecal banks in the US and people lining up to get paid for donating their stool is only the tip of the this new era in the lives of human being "human and gut microbiome symbiosis".

Sadly as the practicing medical professions and specialists are always reluctant to utilize cutting edge science until very large promising RCT data published; we keep prescribing antibiotics as it is the cure of all conditions from throat infection to lyme disease!

Thank to the books like this and relentless efforts of survivors of autoimmune disorders, worried patients often supressed by their doctor would seek the help of their fellow sufferers in the search for an answer. This book has a wealth of knowledge and takes us back to the basics of eating and cooking like our "hunter gatherer" ancestors, as we should have in the first place; After all "We are what we eat".

Dr. Ali Eghtesadi Araghi, MD
Board Certified Metabolic & Nutritional
Medicine (FMMI/ABARRM)

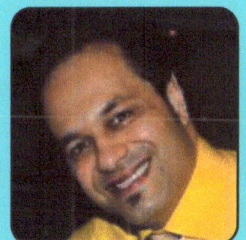

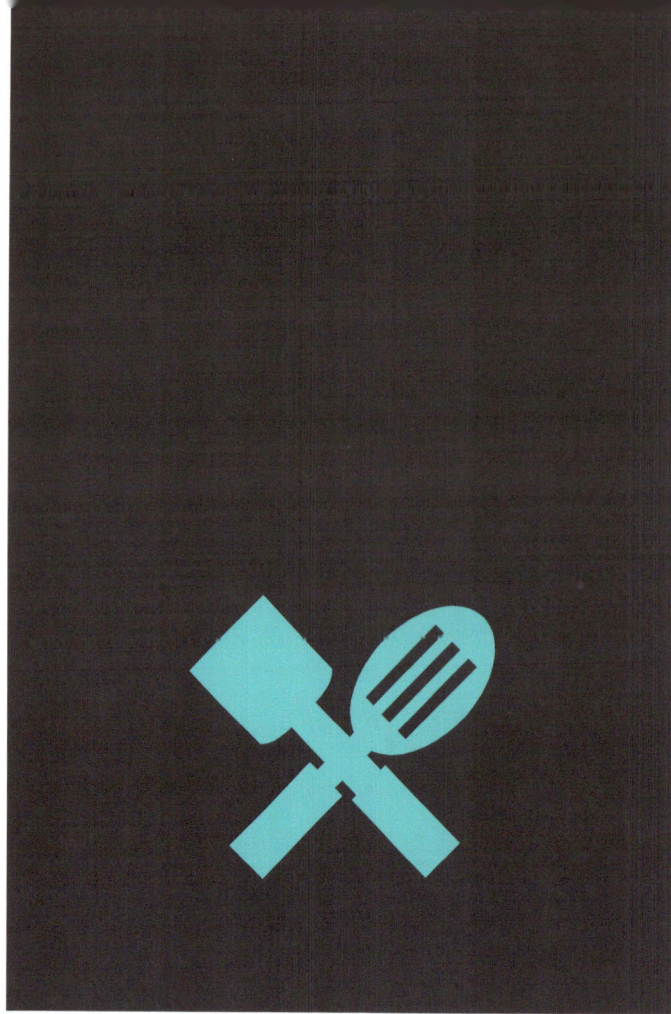

Table of contents

Devotion

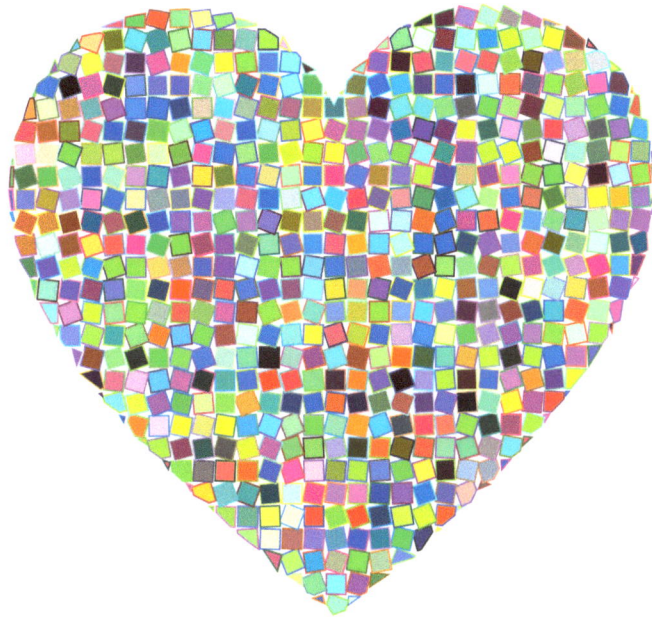

I devote this book to all the people who have autoimmune or other chronic diseases, who like me, are warriors in the pursuit of holistic healing through food and lifestyle. You have given yourself an invaluable gift by taking the leap of faith and reading this book, and embarking on your own Hunt for Harmony: You are a Harmony Hunter!!

Special devotion: To my wonderful husband Stephen and my son Aden for your unwavering support and understanding throughout this adventure. Stephen your patience knows no bounds; it has been a bumpy ride over the past 20 years! I know there were many times that you thought "this isn't what I signed up for!" but you have stuck by me through thick and thin. There is no way I would be where I am today without your unconditional love and support.

My precious son Aden, you are the reason I found my inner strength to keep going no matter how hard it gets. The love you have shown me has humbled me, despite having a very sick Mumma a lot of the time in your young life. You have wrapped your little arms around my neck and kissed my cheeks, looked into my eyes and told me everything will be ok. "You'll get better Mumma! I know you will! Aden, you make me a better person every single day. You are the reason I kept putting one foot in front of the other even when I thought I couldn't; my love for you knows no bounds!

A special thank you to two of the most inspiring friends I have had the honour of knowing. Ashley and Heather Dionysius, and their company AD Marketing, is behind the success of Harmony Hunter. Heather, you have become such a beautiful friend to me and an inspirational autoimmune warrior. As the first person I met who followed a paleo lifestyle, you were the one who sparked my interest in studying paleo and therefore coming across AIP. This book exists because of you!! You have been in my mind's eye as I have created this book. I hope you enjoy cooking the dishes you helped inspire. Ashley, your creative and marketing genius is astounding and this whole project wouldn't be what it is without your expertise. I cannot thank you both enough for your incredible generosity, constant encouragement and support throughout this project. It wouldn't be the success it is without you both!!

I'd also like to take this opportunity to thank Mark and Daniel Rotolone, Cosima Diana, Carlos Ortega and the rest of the Vine Restaurant family for the invaluable knowledge I gained whilst working with you. I learnt so much from all of you; invaluable skills, knowledge and the love of feeding people delicious food! Thank you!!

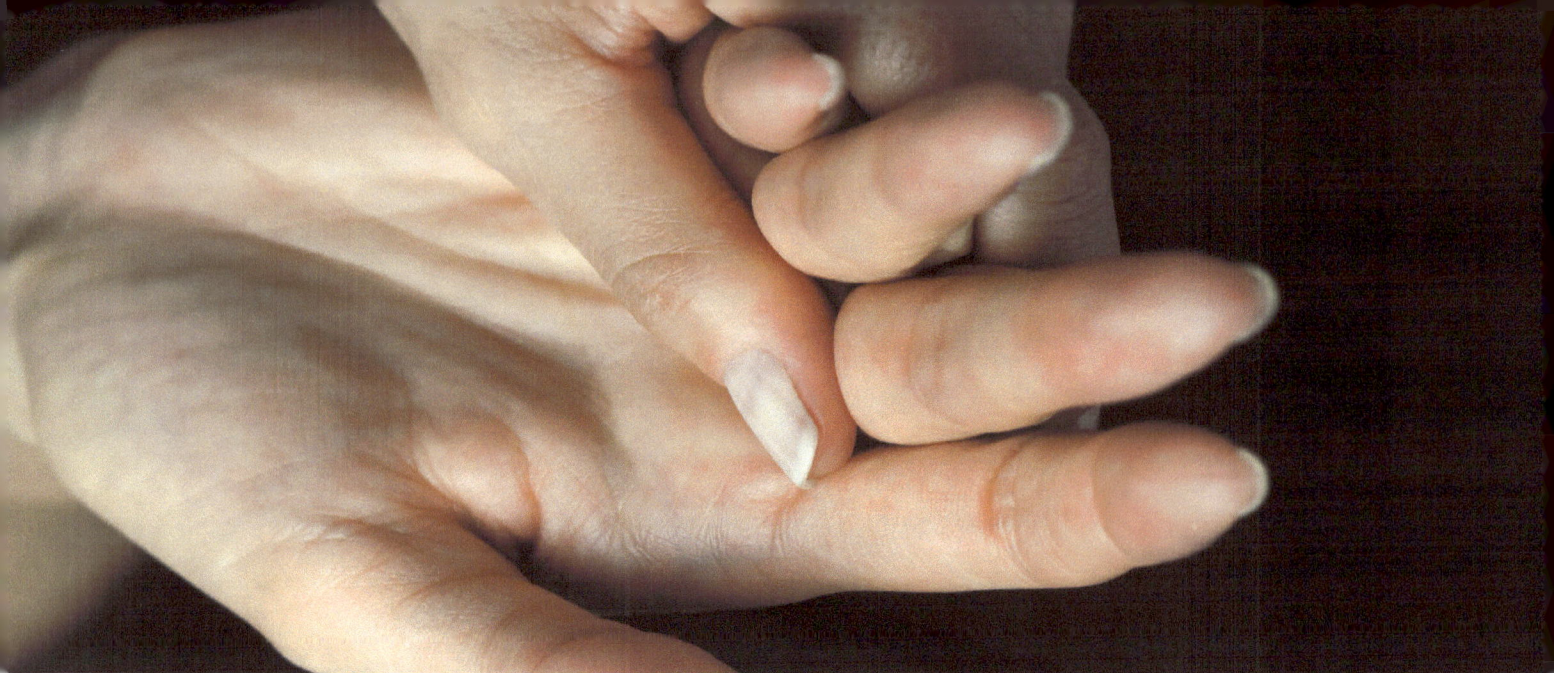

What is the Autoimmune Protocol (AIP)

In a nut free shell, the Autoimmune Protocol is a style of eating that eliminates possible inflammatory foods for deep gut healing of leaky gut (gut symbiosis). The Protocol will reduce inflammation within the body, so that your body can heal. All autoimmune and chronic diseases are caused by a leaky gut, and the resulting immune response triggers that cause your symptoms. By removing these foods you are taking away the triggers that are causing your disease and symptoms, and finally allowing your immune system, gut, body and mind, the time to calm and gently heal itself.

In addition to the regular paleo exclusions you will also be eliminating all nuts, seeds and seed spices including coffee and cacao, eggs, and the nightshade family of vegetables and spices. These foods can be possible allergens or cause an inflammatory impact on the gut and immune system. It is really important for you to focus on the foods you can have and not the foods you can't; you are giving yourself an incredible gift by embarking on this lifestyle of healing.

The recommended time period to be on the AIP is 90 days, subject to how much damage your body has endured and how much healing needs to take place. This isn't about rushing through this process to get back to your old ways of eating; this is a way of life. For me and many others this involves a grieving process of letting go of how we ate before the AIP, as so much of our sense of self, family, traditions and culture revolves around how we nourish our bodies.

For those who are starting reintroductions, this timeline may be shorter or longer, depending on how much gut healing is needed. It will also be due to the level of inflammation your body needs to recover from. The intent is to then reintroduce foods very slowly through a strict staged reintroduction protocol, so you can observe how your body responds. If you introduce a food and subsequently have a reaction, then your body is telling you that you are not yet ready to incorporate this food back into your diet.

This is not to say that you will never be able to reintroduce that food again, although this might well be the case. You can keep trying further down the road after more healing has taken place. Many people are able to successfully reintroduce all eliminated foods, whereas some may only be able to reintroduce some foods, or only eat certain foods occasionally.

Don't be disheartened! This is totally normal. Be focused on how your body has healed and feels. It is a really important concept of AIP to really learn to listen to your body. It is an incredible machine and it knows what it does and does not need. Too often people continue eating or doing certain things simply because "it's good for you" e.g. like eating kale as it is all the rage now. Just because something may be considered healthy doesn't mean it is the right thing for your body!

An excellent way to track how foods are affecting your body is to start a food/symptom journal. Just write down what you are eating and how it is affecting your body. Document any symptoms you may experience after ingesting certain foods, for example, how is your digestion? Are there symptoms of constipation or diarrhoea, any sinus or mucus production, sneezing or coughing, nausea or vomiting, headaches, brain fog or lack of concentration? Track whether or not you are experiencing insomnia or other sleep difficulties or an increase in anxiety or depression symptoms. Skin irritations or rashes such as hives may occur as the body has adverse immune responses to the foods we are eating. Yes, these symptoms are also probably associated with your illness, which is why it is so important to really learn to listen to what your body is saying to you.

Whilst on the AIP lifestyle journey, a very important factor to take into consideration is the presence of underlying co-infections within the gut and body. These can have an inhibiting effect on your healing and recovery. Helicobacter Pylori, Epstein Barr Syndrome and overgrowth of Candida are some of these co-infections, which may be culprits in affecting the results you want to achieve. Having or finding a good functional integrated medicine doctor and/or relevant holistic practitioners will be invaluable in treating your condition/s in a more holistic way. Check out the Australian College of Environmental and Nutritional Medicine https://www.acnem.org/find-a-practitioner or the Mindd Foundation http://mindd.org/practitioners/practitioners-search/ to help you find the right practitioner for your needs.

Foods to permanently remove from your menu are:

- All refined vegetable oils including canola and cottonseed.
- Legumes including soy and peanuts.
- All grains including corn.
- Refined cane sugars, sugar alcohols such as mannitol, zylitol and processed stevia.
- Thickeners, emulsifiers, any preservatives and artificial additives of any kind.
- All processed foods.

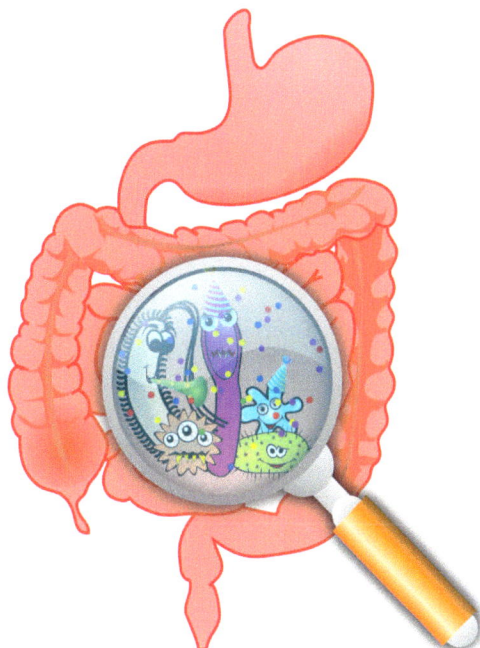

About Autoimmune Disease

Autoimmune disease is a very serious disorder affecting millions of people worldwide. The disease can be difficult to diagnose for medical practitioners due to their wide variety. There are more than 80 different types that are known and many more are being discovered; or in some cases diseases are being re-classified as autoimmune.

Treatment options mainly focus on relief, as there are currently no curative therapies available; however it is possible to put these conditions into remission following AIP. Sadly many people are misdiagnosed with a plethora of other conditions, as autoimmune symptoms mimic many other conditions such as mental health issues. Many patients spend years being misdiagnosed and often treated with medicine or other therapies which can actually exacerbate their conditions, before they finally get a true diagnosis. They are then left with the unenviable task of trying to recover from their misdiagnosis, while often embarking on treatment protocols that miss one of the biggest issue of autoimmune disease, gut dysbiosis or leaky gut.

An important part of the treatment is to eat a healthy balanced diet. Autoimmune Protocol Paleo is designed to provide followers with healthy, tasty and nutritious recipes, whilst avoiding foods known to cause inflammation within the body and leaky gut, which causes autoimmunity. In addition to following the AIP, implementing strategies to manage stress are essential. Introducing mindfulness, self care routines and light exercise, such as yoga, to your daily routine, will allow your body to calm and gently heal.

When you have been diagnosed with an autoimmune disease and decide to embark on the AIP journey, you will almost immediately discover that 'regular' ready-made foods such as pre-prepared sauces, marinades and other processed convenience foods are off the list. This is a hard concept for many people as our lives have become so busy, and most people are time poor and have become reliant on convenience foods. You need to take a different look at what food, cooking and eating means to you. This is a chance also for you to reconnect with how you nourish your body, and where your food comes from, instead of going for the quickest but least nutrient dense options. You have to start cooking for yourself in a totally different manner than you may have been used to.

Not an easy task for many.

It is my intention to help you get going in the kitchen, and discover how wonderfully satisfying it is creating delicious, nutrient dense dishes from scratch, that not only nourish your body but your soul as well!

We have sadly become quite disconnected from our food, where it comes from, who grows it, how it is grown, how animals are raised. It is an integral part of the AIP and Paleo lifestyle to reconnect to how we nurture and nourish our bodies.

"Every time you eat or drink you are either feeding disease or fighting it"- Heather Morgan

I am here to provide you with a comprehensive set of recipes that I have created along my AIP journey, designed with Australian seasonal produce and lifestyle in mind. I will be familiarizing you with some kitchen basics that will help you unleash your inner chef, and give you the confidence you need to be the master of your kitchen.

I want you to go on a culinary adventure with your AIP journey. To have fun experimenting with different flavours and recipes you may have never tried. I want you to add your own personal stamp on your food, by adding different herbs and spices, or simply adding more or less of an ingredient. Just because the recipe says how much you will need to add doesn't mean it is set in stone. Yes, sometimes things don't work out how you would have expected, but that's ok! It is all part of embracing this new lifestyle and healing your body. Above all I want you to have fun with the food you are creating and healing your body with.

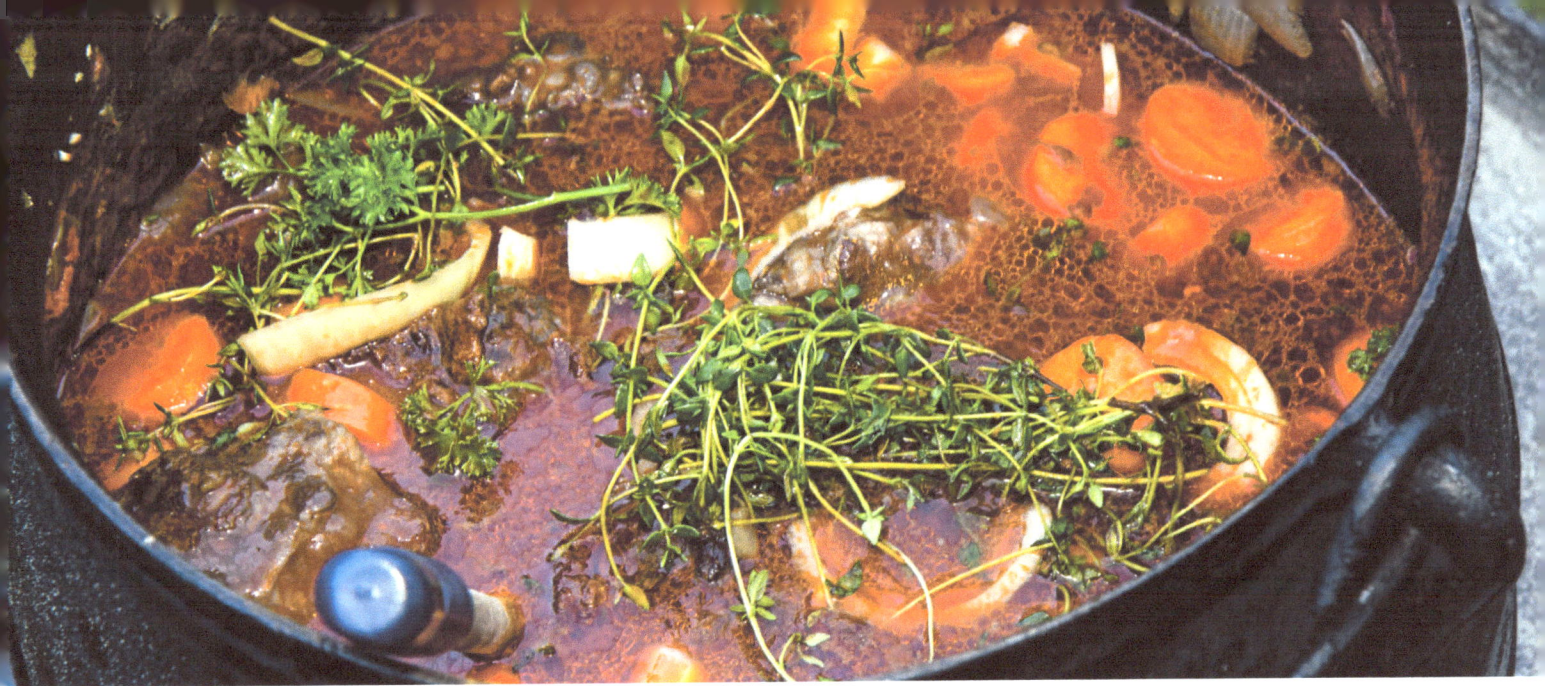

A word on batch cooking

Batch cooking is a fantastic way to make sure you have a good supply of prepared food on hand; this is not only cost effective but will save you time and energy in the long run. The basic principle behind batch cooking is to think like a chef. Any a la carte restaurant you go to have the components of your dish prepared well in advance before you even order your meal. When an order comes into the kitchen the chefs aren't preparing your dish from scratch or you would be waiting a very long time for your meal! This is how you need to think of the food you're preparing. This isn't as difficult as it may sound; all it will take is a little preparation and setting aside enough time to prepare your meals. On average I will set aside 4-5 hours a week for batch cooking.

Firstly, you will need to choose the meals you want to cook, and decide if you want to double, or even triple, a recipe, ensuring you have enough fridge/freezer space. Once you have decided what meals you are going to cook, make a list of all the ingredients you will need. A really good tip is to choose dishes with common ingredients in them. By doing this you will not only save money by not having to buy too many different ingredients, but also save on prepping time.

The next consideration is utilising all available cooking methods at your disposal. For example, when I batch cook I have the oven going with all of the racks being used, the slow cooker going and also use all the burners on my stove. This may sound daunting at first, but with a little practice and organisation you will be batching like a pro in no time!

Once you have yourself set up and ready, think about what you are cooking and the times and methods you'll need to make your dishes. For example you're going to cook a bone broth, a lamb shank curry, and roasted root vegetable salad with marinated chicken.
First step is to get your oven hot, then salt your bones and shanks on separate trays then into the oven to brown for the specified time. While they are in the oven get your slow cooker warming up, then prep the vegies for the broth, curry and salad.

Get your vegies for the broth in the slow cooker and add remaining ingredients to the slow cooker for your broth. Set aside the vegies for the curry and if you have another rack or two in the oven get your vegies in the oven for your salad.

Once all those are cooking away, set about getting the remainder of the components of your dishes ready such as the spice mix of your curry, marinading the chicken and the dressing for the salad.

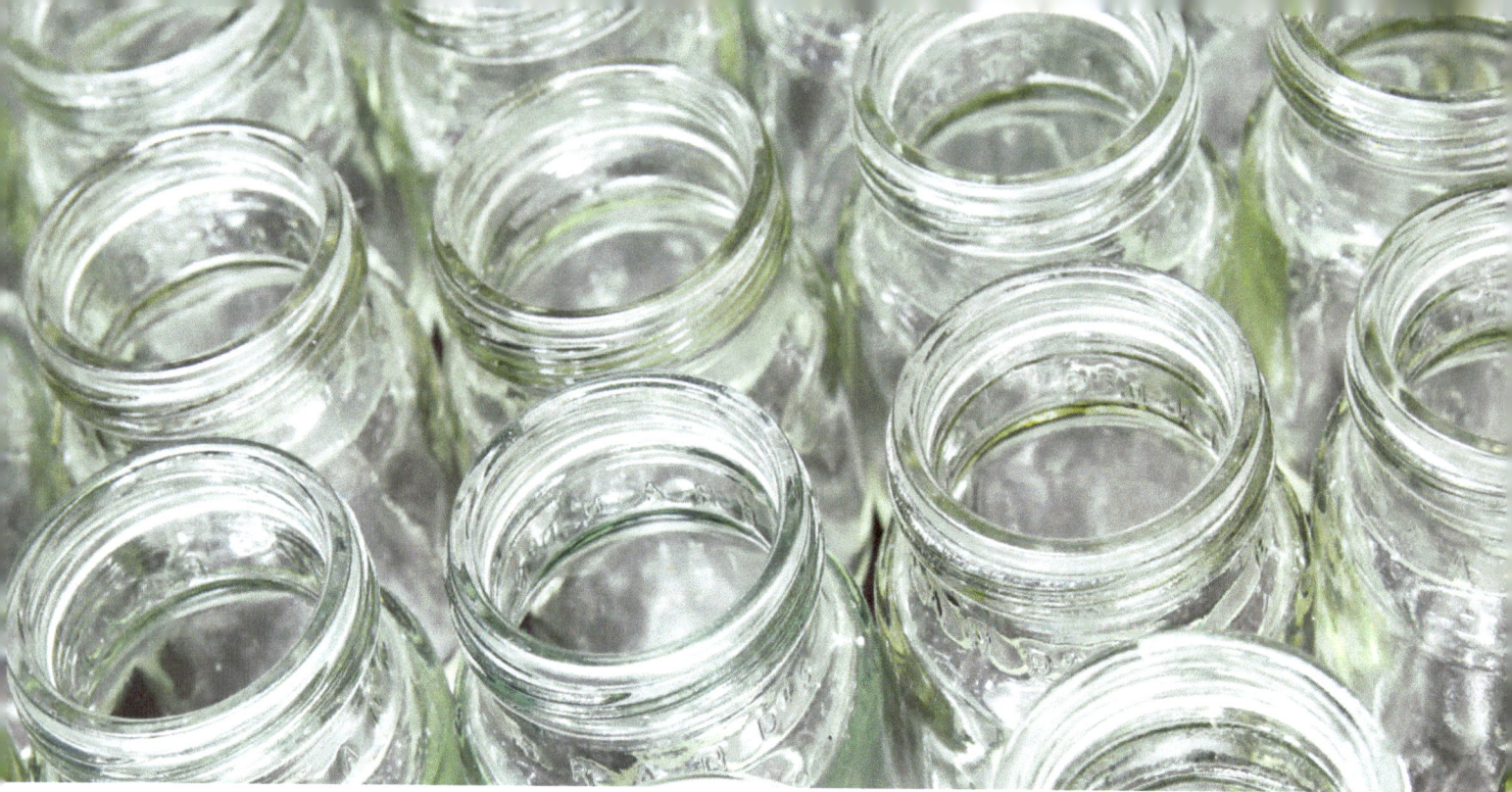

A word on batch cooking

When your bones and meat are nice and brown you can get on to putting the last of the broth on, and curry together. A good tip, so as not to lose all the wonderful caramelised bits on the roasting trays, is to pour a bit of boiling water in the trays, allowing to sit for a minute or two, then use a spatula to scrape up the browned bits and add them to your dishes.

When your vegies are done, set them aside to cool and fry up your chicken thighs. Then you will have a beautiful gut healing broth, a warming curry for dinners and a mixed veggie salad with a great source of protein for lunches to get you through the week!

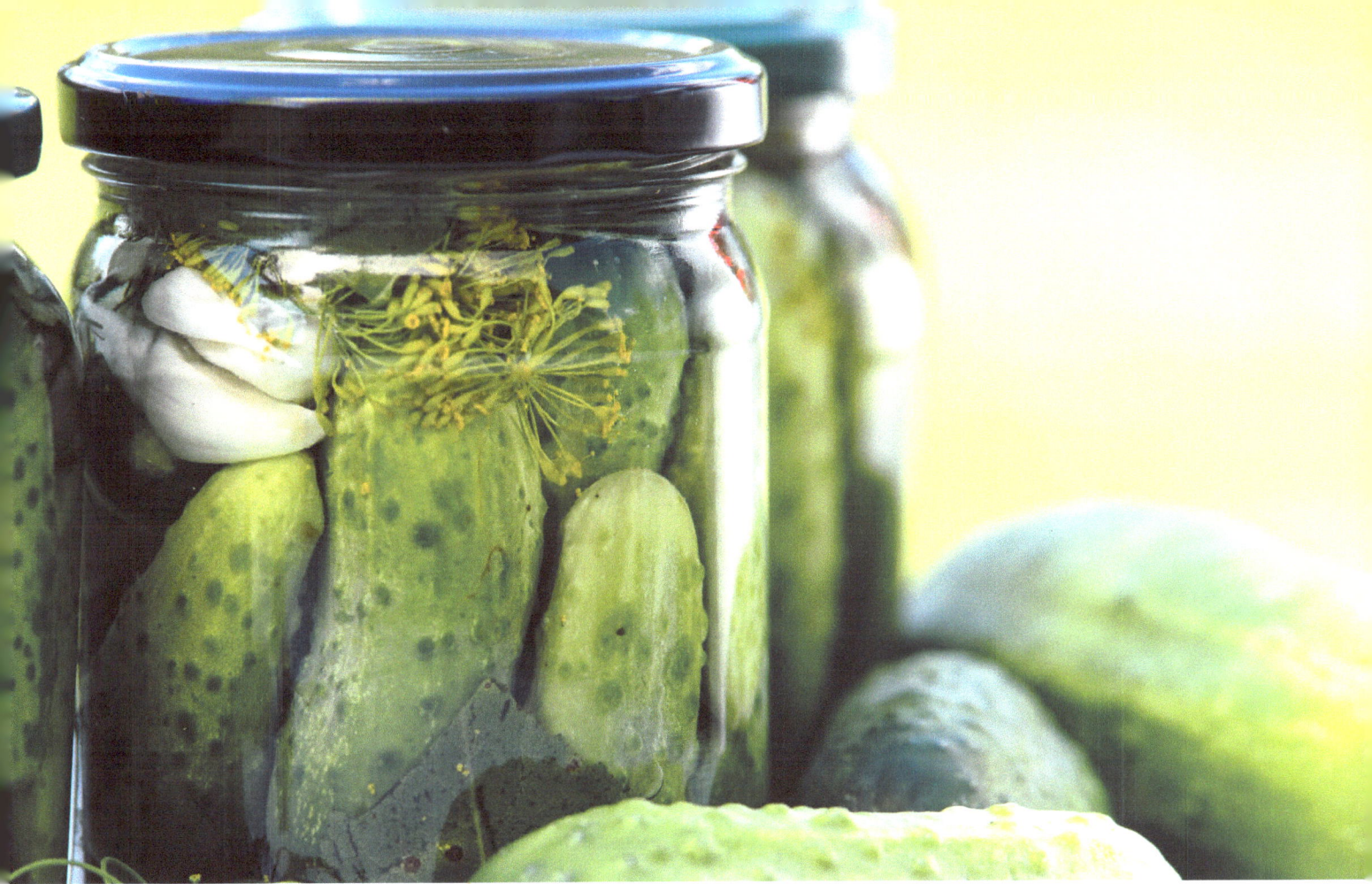

Fermented Vegetables and Drinks

Fermented foods have been a part of people's diets for thousands of years. This is not only because the fermenting process preserves perishable foods, but also because they are very high in gut friendly probiotics and easily absorbable vitamins and minerals. They can be a very beneficial aspect of healing leaky gut as they are very high in gut friendly bacteria that helps restore the balance of good bacteria in the gut. This has a huge impact on strengthening the immune system.

There are literally hundreds, if not thousands, of different types of ferments you can make and buy. From the world famous - sauerkraut and yogurt, to the more recently popular kombucha and kefir.

I believe that fermented vegetables play a crucial role in the AIP lifestyle but some caution should be exercised when choosing to consume fermented beverages such as kombucha and kefir. These can be high in sugar and the yeast that is present in these ferment cultures can have a negative effect on the gut if there is underlying overgrowth of Candida or SIBO (small intestinal bacterial overgrowth) for example. The yeasts and sugars in these drinks can actually have the reverse effect by feeding the overgrowth and making symptoms worse.

So in summary, yes ferments are important to include in your diet. Add a good spoonful of fermented veggies to each meal to enrich your diet with good probiotics, vitamins and minerals. Just be sure that you don't have any underlying co-infections that these foods or drinks may aggravate.

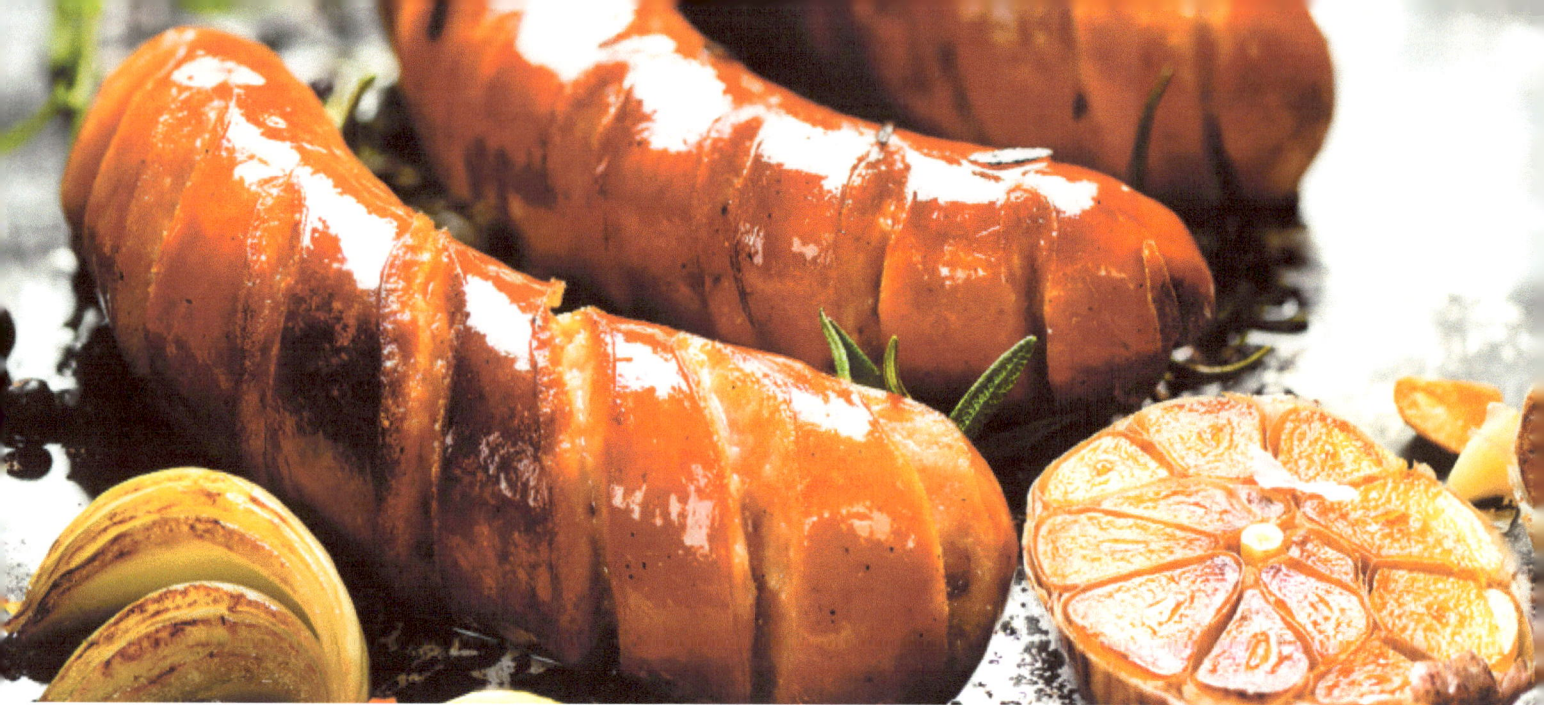

Breakfasts on AIP

When you start on AIP, breakfasts are going to be very different to what you may have been eating for most of your life, in most cases. Gone are the grains that make up the vast majority of people's breakfasts. Many people are getting hunger pangs within a short time after breakfast, and will often go for a sweet snack before lunch as their blood sugar drops. This is simply because they are not fuelling their body with enough nutrient density and protein to get through the morning. As I have mentioned you will need to embrace a whole new way of eating, and break the cycle of consuming foods that have contributed to your illness. With a little practice and thought your old breakfasts will become a distant memory, and you'll wonder how you managed before!

Here are a few examples of how your AIP breakfast may look:-

•   Leftovers from the night before

•   AIP brekkie fry ups with vitamin rich livers, your favourite veggies sautéed in good quality fat, served with bacon, avocado and a lemon wedge

•   Soups or stews

•   Smoothies, your favourite blend with a tablespoon or two of grass fed collagen powder for a protein punch, with added gut healing benefits

•   Meat patties cooked up ahead of time and thawed in the fridge overnight to be reheated under the grill, for example. Also add lots of veggies to your patties too!!

•   Always have a good tablespoon or two of fermented vegetables with each meal for a good hit of gut healing friendly bacteria and vitamins!

•   A mug of bone broth on the side of your breakfasts, or any meal for that matter, is great for a protein hit and has amazing deep gut healing properties.

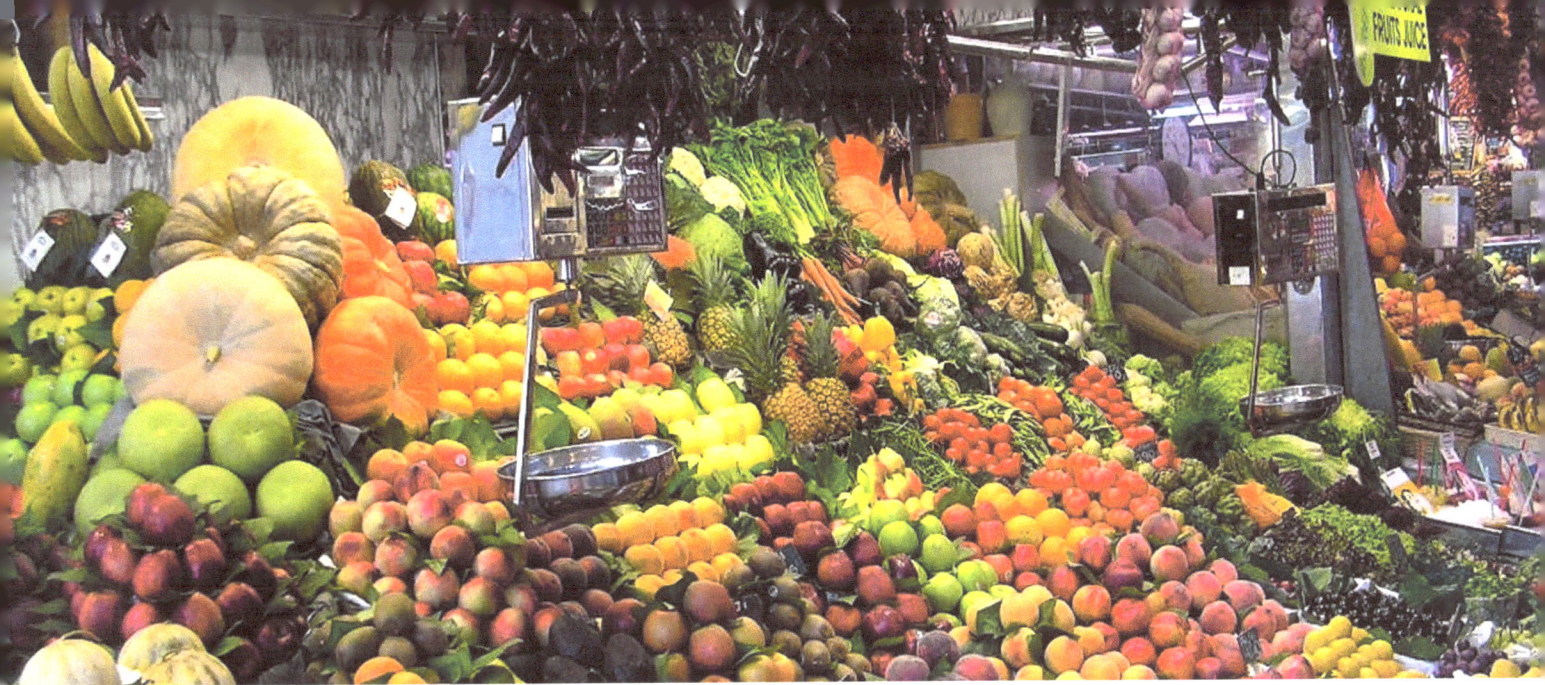

Shopping Tips and Tricks

Before you even start AIP, work out where you are going to source your food. Is it going to be from local farmers' markets, local co-op, local green grocers, local butchers or the supermarket? Notice I used the word local a lot? This is because it is not only great to support and get to know your local producers, but it will ensure you are getting the freshest produce available, as in most cases the food has been grown or raised within your local area. Supermarkets, as you may know, tend to store fresh food including eggs, for in some cases many months!!! This sadly means that a lot of the nutrient quality has been lost or not even properly developed because produce is harvested green and unripened, to help prevent loss to pests in the field or increase the time the produce can be stored. Another great reason to shop from local producers is you will save money!!

Produce from markets etc will be, in the majority of cases, cheaper than buying from big supermarket chains. If for a variety of reasons you are unable to shop from local producers this is totally fine, don't fret!! Eating the AIP paleo way is a far more nutrient dense way to eat than eating a heavily processed diet, devoid of nutrition and healing. Eating a heavily processed diet is the biggest contributor to chronic disease in our society today and we are exponentially getting sicker as a community every year because of this.

Go organic or not organic? Yes, it far better to buy organic for many reasons - no chemical sprays and fertilisers, less chemicals for your body to contend with, less impact to the environment, better soil quality, thus increasing nutrient density, and in many cases improved shelf life. The animals are raised in a much more respected and high quality environment and are not exposed to hormones, antibiotics and steroids.

This will mean less of these nasties make their way into your body causing inflammation and chronic diseases.

Another big factor to consider is the exposure to GMOs. There is overwhelming evidence on the negative health impacts of consuming these franken foods. You may have noticed an increasing number of imported fresh produce on the shelves of supermarkets in the last decade or so. Many of these foods come from countries that heavily cultivate GMO crops and there are still no labelling laws to disclose whether or not GMO practices have been used. Also, many of the brands of processed foods that we have often grown up with, or have known and trusted, are actually owned and produced by global biotech, or big food companies. These companies extensively use GMO ingredients and other chemical additives in their products to ensure high profits for their shareholders. This also means cheap prices for the consumer and "food" devoid of any nutrition that causes people to become addicted to their products, and contributes to chronic diseases.

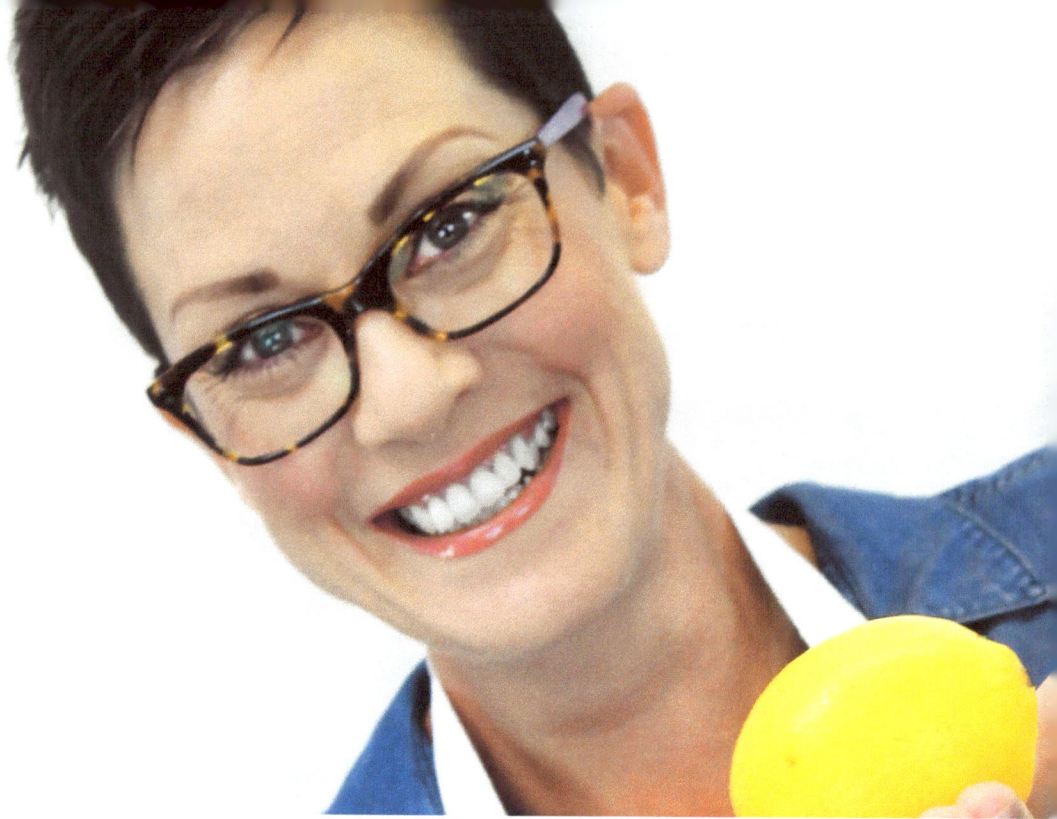

Seasonal produce is another important factor to consider. Buying seasonally will not only be cheaper, it will be more nutritionally dense than imported produce that has been in storage for long periods of time and travelled for thousands of kilometres.

Another great tip is to find out when the specials are on and when mark downs are made on fresh produce. Buying seconds are another great example where you can save money. Often at markets, green grocers or supermarkets, they will do bulk deals on items such as carrots in large lots because they are broken, odd shaped or marked. There is nothing wrong with this food, it still has the same nutrients. It may be less appealing to the eye, but you can save yourself a lot of money looking out for these specials. Talk to your local stall holders or shop keepers and ask them when they take delivery of fresh stock and mark down older stock. This also applies to meat, find out when the mark downs are on and save yourself some money. This is a great tool for batch cooking as well when you see something at a good deal, stock up and whip up a big batch of your favourite dish.

Buying dry goods and pantry items online or creating a small co-op with friends and family is another great way to save money. Often these types of items such as coconut oil, flours, herbs, spices and dried goods are much cheaper when sourced online. This is my preference to buying small quantities from health food shops or supermarkets. Forming a co-op not only shares the cost of buying products in bulk, but creates a sense of community as well. Work out what the common items are that everyone uses, source items in bulk online, and receive great products at a fraction of the retail cost!

My Nan always said, "Look after the pennies and the pounds will take care of themselves"

Eating out while on the AIP lifestyle

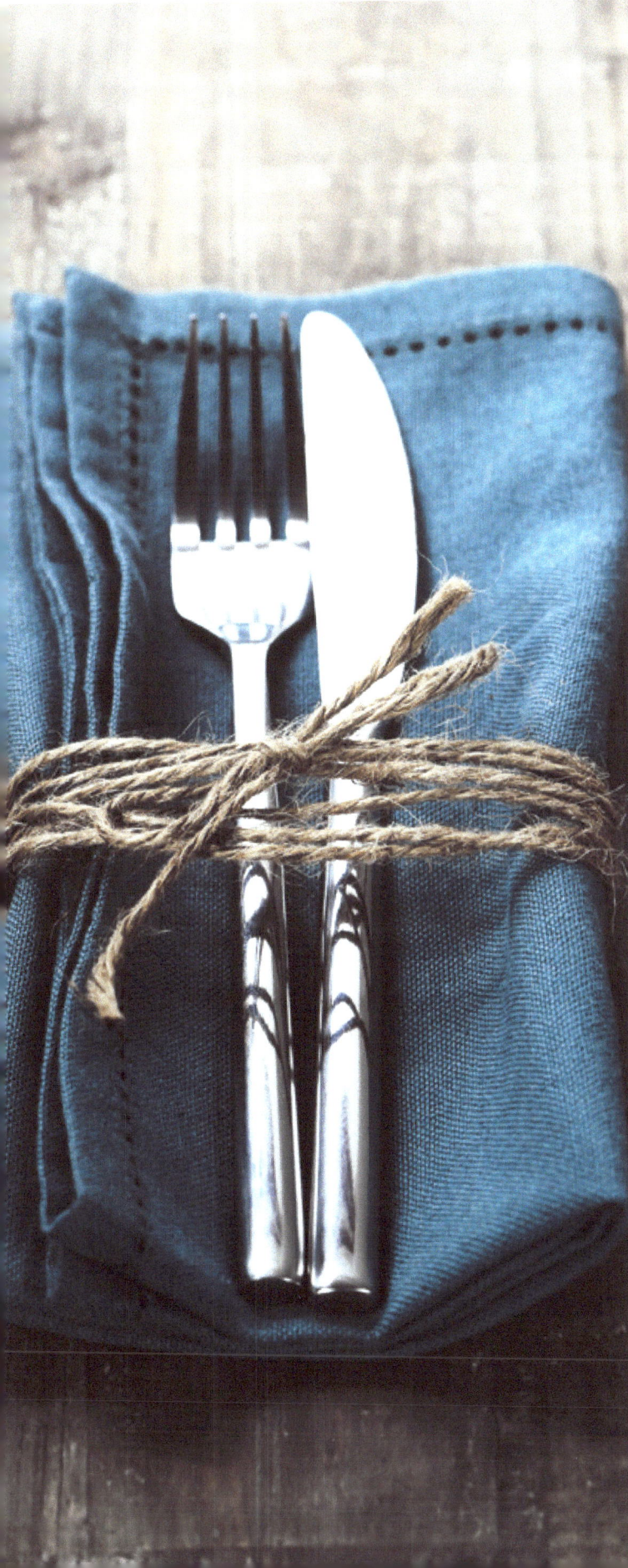

Eating out on AIP doesn't have to be difficult with a little fore thought and preparation. We are lucky enough now to have many paleo and whole foods style cafes and restaurants popping up, as this way of life gains popularity and momentum. However you will need to be mindful when ordering out to not expose yourself to possible foods that aren't AIP friendly. Simply make sure you are very familiar with the approved foods and always ask when ordering if you are unsure. So often a substitution or removal of a particular component is possible. Another important question to ask is the types of oils, sauces or dressings that are used as often they are not AIP friendly; so you could, for example, ask for a simple oil and vinegar dressing.

Taking my own food with me is how I mostly 'eat out'. It is more cost effective and there are no worries about having to recover from possible food contamination. If you do not have one or more already, invest in a wide mouth thermos, which can keep food hot or cold for up to twelve hours. I like having the wide mouth option as you can take the whole top off easily to eat soups or stews, or even a cold salad! Another way of transporting cold foods is a good quality insulated lunch box. There are so many on offer, however my favourite, which I have been using for many years since pre-AIP, are the Fridge-To-Go insulated lunch bags. There are several size options from small through to picnic sized, but their magic lies within the specially designed slim cooling blocks that are removable. These surround the food on all sides, literally keeping food cool for up to 8 hours. Now in our Aussie hot summers these are a fantastic investment!

Reduction of Chemical Exposure from personal care, household items and even water

Something that is often over looked when taking a holistic approach to healing and addressing chronic diseases; is the exposure to chemicals in personal care products, household items and even the water that comes from our tap. They are in everything and we have been led to believe for decades that these chemicals are safe and harmless and that couldn't be further from the truth!

We are being exposed to an ever increasing array of toxic poisons that are contributing greatly to chronic disease; putting enormous strain on our immune system and detoxification pathways, and inhibiting the ability to heal and recover. Many companies are waking up to the fact that consumers are becoming aware of the detrimental effects of the use of these poisons. Sadly they are marketing and labelling many products as 'natural' or 'contains natural or organic ingredients'. However many of these products still contain toxic poisons. Many people are unaware of how many products are in the home that contains these toxic chemicals that we use several times daily.

Our drinking water is another potential source of exposure to toxic chemicals such as chlorine and fluoride. Fluoridation of our drinking water has been a hot button topic for a long time now, and there are numerous studies that prove that fluoride causes detrimental health problems. There are many water filter options available to suit any budget. Another important factor to consider is making sure the system you choose also alkalises your water. Pure clean alkaline water is essential to good health. There are also filters available you can fit to your bath, shower or your whole home.

Removing these products from your life will take a huge load off your body and help you heal. There is an amazing selection of natural personal care and household products now available, at very affordable prices. These are not only healthier for you and environmentally safe, but they are far more effective than their toxic chemical counterparts. .

Personal care items that contain toxic chemicals;

- Toothpaste, mouthwashes and dental flosses
- Shampoos, conditioners, styling products, hair dyes
- Body washes, soaps, body scrubs
- Deodorants, perfumes and body sprays
- Facial cleansers, scrubs, moisturisers, masks
- Make up, make up removers, nail polish and removers
- Sunscreen, self tanners and bronzers
- Personal insect repellents

Household products that contain toxic chemicals

- Dish washing liquids, dish washer powders and tablets, rinse aids
- Surface cleaning sprays, window cleaning sprays, stainless steel cleaners, oven cleaners, floor washes
- Bathroom cleaners, cream cleansers, mould killer sprays, bleach, toilet cleaners, drain cleaners
- Air freshener sprays and diffusers, fragrance candles, fragranced oils
- Laundry detergents, stain removers, laundry soakers, fabric softeners, ironing sprays
- Insect killing sprays, surface sprays and powders, insect baits and bombs
- Garden pest sprays and fertilisers, weed control products.

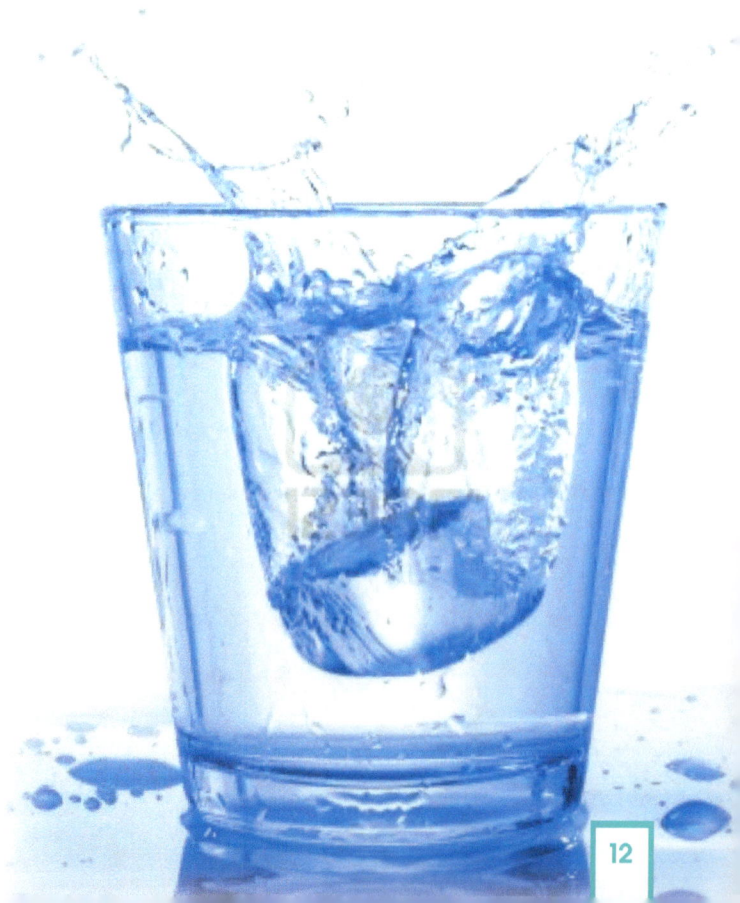

The shopping ingredients list for the AIP lifestyle

There is no cooking without ingredients! Your kitchen should have a number of dry and wet spices plus ingredients that you will likely use on a daily basis.

I strongly suggest that before you start you cleanse your kitchen of non AIP/Paleo ingredients. It will make it a lot easier to avoid temptation from eliminated foods, if they are not on hand. If the thought of wasting good food bothers you, perhaps you could donate any unwanted food to your local food bank or relevant charities. Even though these foods may no longer be desirable to you, there are many people that would greatly appreciate them in a time of need.

Below is a comprehensive list of all the approved AIP foods.

VEGETABLES	ROOT VEGETABLES	FRUIT		FATS
Artichoke	Beetroot	Apple	Persimmon	Avocado Oil
Rocket	Celery	Apricot	Plum	Animal Fat
Asparagus	Carrot	Avocado	Pineapple	Coconut Oil
Bok Choi	Onion	Banana	Pomegranate	Duck Fat
Broccoli	Parsnip	Blackberry	Raspberry	Lard
Brussel Sprout	Turnip	Blueberry	Strawberry	Olive Oil
Cabbage	Rutabaga	Rockmelon	Tangerine	Sustainably Sourced
Cauliflower	Radish	Cherry	Watermelon	Palm Oil
Celery	Shallot	Clementine		
Silver Beet	Sweet Potato	Coconut		
Collard Green	Yam	Date		
Cucumber	Spring Onions	Fig		
Fennel		Grape		
Kale		Grapefruit		
Leek		Guava		
Lettuce		Huckleberry		
Mushroom		Honeydew		
Rhubarb		Kiwi		
Spinach		Lemon		
Squash		Lime		
Watercress		Mango		
Pumpkin		Marionberry		
		Nectarine		
		Orange		
		Papaya		
		Peach		
		Pear		

MEATS	OFFAL'S	HERBS	SPICES	FERMENTS	STANDARD PANTRY ITEMS
Beef	Bone Broth	Basil	Cinnamon	Fermented Vegetables	Apple-cider Vinegar
Lamb	Liver	Bay Leaves	Cloves	Kombucha	Anchovies
Fish	Kidney	Chamomile	Garlic	Water Kefir	Arrowroot Powder
Shellfish	Heart	Chives	Ginger	Sauerkraut	Coconut Flour
Chicken	Brains	Coriander	Saffron	Carrot	Coconut Flakes
Turkey		Dill	Pink Salt	Beetroot	Coconut Vinegar
Duck		Lavender	Shallots	Other Veggies	Coconut Aminos
Pork		Lemongrass	Turmeric		Dates
		Marjoram			Dried Fruit
		Mint			Olives
		Parsley			Salmon
		Peppermint			Sardines
		Rosemary			Tuna
		Sage			Umeplum Vinegar
		Spearmint			Banana Flour
		Tarragon			Raw Honey
		Thyme	Rapudura	Coconut Sugar	Pure Maple Syrup

You will not need all of this at one go, base the purchases you make on a weekly meal plan and buy only what is needed.

This is the list of foods to avoid.

SEEDS	EGGS	NIGHTSHADES	BEANS & LEGUMES	GRAINS	DAIRY	NUTS
Anise	Chicken	Cayenne	Adzuki Beans	Amaranth	Butter	Almond
Cacao	Duck	Chilli Pepper	Black Beans	Barley	Cheese	Brazil
Caraway	Goose	Eggplant	Black-eyed Peas	Buckwheat	Cream	Hazelnut
Chia		Goji Berry	Chickpeas	Bulgur	Cream Cheese	Pecan
Coriander		Ground Cherry	Fava Beans	Corn	Ghee	Macadamia
Cumin		Habañero	Lentils	Farro	Milk	Walnut
Fennel Seed		Jalapeño	Lima Beans	Kamut	Yogurt	
Fenugreek		Paprika	Peanuts	Millet		
Mustard		Poblano	Kidney Beans	Oats		
Nutmeg		Potato	Soybeans	Quinoa		
Poppy		Sweet Pepper		Rice		
Pumpkin		Tobacco		Rye		
Sesame		Tomato		Sorghum		
Sunflower		Tomatillo		Spelt		
Hemp		Wolf Berries		Teff		
Coffee				Wheat		

List of Recipes

THE BASICS

SOUPS

SALADS

SEAFOODS

POULTRY

MEAT

List of Recipes

OFFALS

DESSERTS

SMOOTHIES

THE BASICS

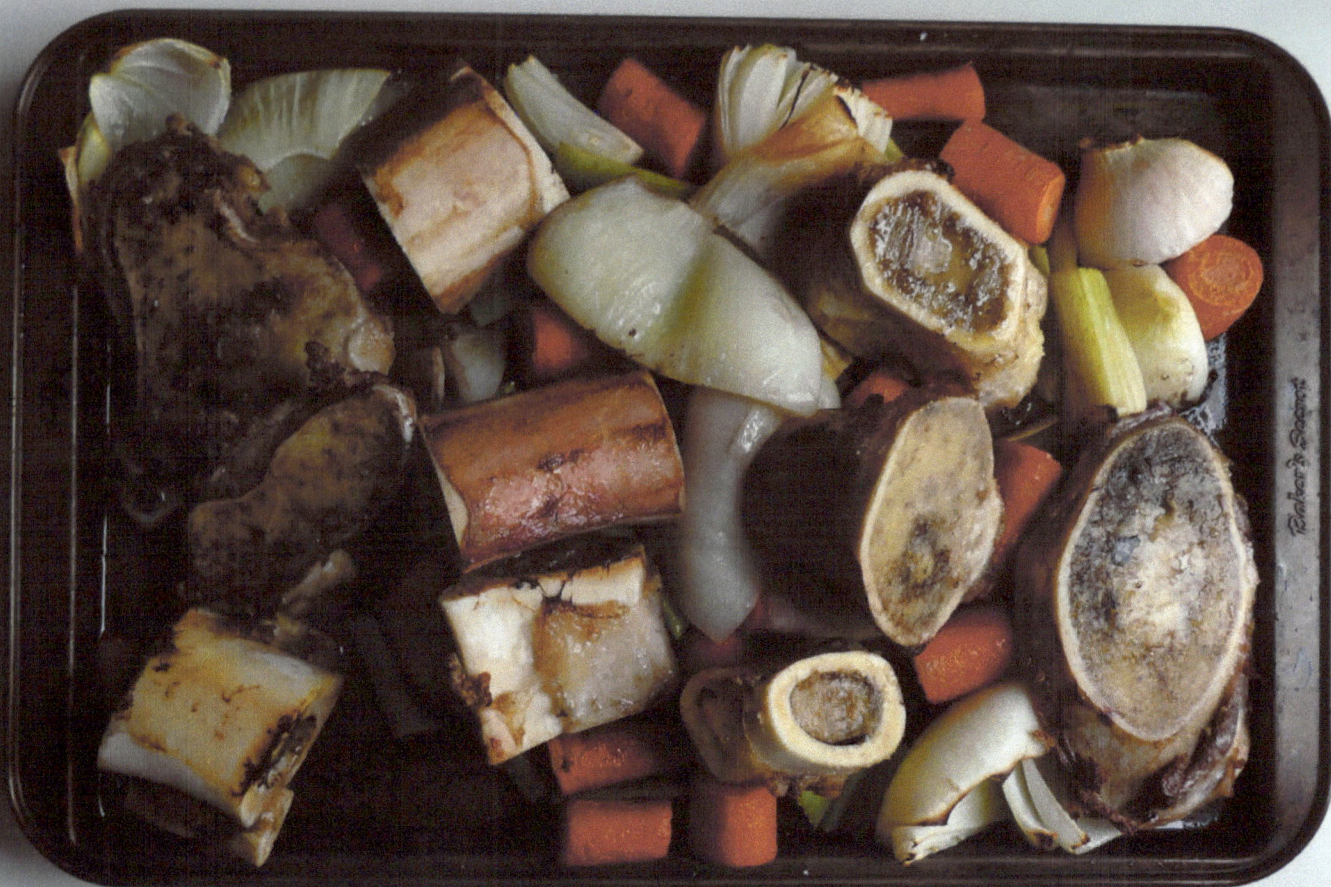

THE ESSENTIAL BONE BROTH

Bone broths are an integral staple in the AIP and Paleo lifestyle, and are considered a super food for their amazing healing properties. Very high in easily absorbable vitamins and minerals and glycine and proline, these crucial nutrients are essentially the glue that holds our bodies together. Bone broth plays a vital role in helping heal leaky gut by repairing the micro damage that has been done. They are also anti-inflammatory and aid in reducing immune response, therefore turn inhibiting the activation of inflammatory cells in your body.

There are a few different cooking method options available when making broth. These include a large capacity slow cooker, a pressure cooker, the latest instant pot, or simply on the stove top. The smartest idea here is to be able to make a large enough batch relatively easily, so you have a constant supply of this amazing healing elixir. It is perfect to drink at breakfast, add to your soups, stews and curries, just to name a few.

When making broths it is important to experiment with different combinations of bones from different animals, however you can stick with the one animal if you prefer. For example you can mix beef and lamb bones together, you may be using beef bones but you can easily add in a few roasted lamb neck chops or shanks as well. When the meat is tender you can remove the meat from the bones then return the bones to the pot so they can continue to leach out their wonderful goodness. By adding a duck frame to a chicken broth you can add an amazing depth of flavour.

The types of bones are a very important thing to consider as well. The bones that have a lot of collagen and cartilage, such as necks, backs, joints, trotters, chicken feet, tails, marrow bones etc, will impart more of their nutrients to your finished broth. Don't be put off by the thought of using these parts of the animal as they are purely there for their incredible healing properties and you will not taste them in the finished product. If you have large bones such as marrow, ask your butcher to saw them up for you.

I highly recommend roasting your bones, meaty bits, and vegetables first before you add them to the Broth; with the exception of roasting the bones for a fish broth or stock. This roasting process will give a much richer depth of flavour and colour.

When adding herbs and vegetables to flavour your broth and impart their goodness, it is best to add them in the last couple of hours, when you are using a slow cooker or stove top method. Cooking these aromatics for too long will result in a bitter tasting broth. Likewise for cooking your broth for too long, a general guide is approximately 4-6 hours for poultry, 1 ½ hours for fish based broths and a minimum of 6 plus hours for harder bones from beef etc. The idea is to extract as much from the bones as possible in some cases broths can be cooked for up to 40 hours!

When you have cooked and strained your broth, if it has had the correct length of cooking time, it should set like jelly when refrigerated. You can then scoop off any of the solidified fat and use it for another purpose. Typically, broth can be stored in the fridge for around 5 days, but you can extend this shelf life by bringing the broth back up to a boil. This will kill off any bacteria that may be forming, and give you another 5 days of shelf life. This can be done multiple times or just freeze what you will not be using for another time.

Below I have given you three basic broths to get you started, please feel free to experiment with your own unique flavour profiles.

BEEF BONE BROTH

Preparation time:
10 mins

Cooking time:
2-6 plus hours dependant on cooking method used

Ingredients:

Yields approx 2-3 litres using an 8 litre pot

- 1.5 kg (3lb) organic grass fed beef bones
- 800g (1.1lb) ox tail
- 2 stalks of celery including the leaves roughly chopped
- 2 carrots roughly chopped
- 2 brown onions roughly chopped
- 2 fresh bay leaves

- Whole bulb of garlic smashed with heel of your palm, no need to peel
- Filtered water
- Pink salt
- 2 tbsp apple cider vinegar
- Small bunch of herbs for example thyme, rosemary, parsley or oregano or a combination of your favourite herbs

Method:

1. Preheat your oven to 200 degrees and liberally salt the bones and the ox tail and roast for around 30-40 mins, until well browned. You can also roast your veggies at the same time if you want; just set them aside after roasting if you are using a slow cooker or stove top method.

2. Put the bones into the pot that you are using, and pour some boiling water into the roasting tray. Allow it to stand for a few minutes, then using a spatula scrape up any of the caramelised bits on the bottom of the pan and add this to the pot.

3. If you are using a pressure cooker or instant pot, add the remainder of the ingredients to the pot and top up with water. Cook for manufactures recommended length of time.

4. If using a slow cooker or stove top method add in the apple cider vinegar and top up with water and simmer for preferred amount of time. For the stove top method, bring the bones to a boil then scoop off any scum/foam that appears on the surface, and then reduce heat to a simmer. If you just simmer the bones and don't boil them first you won't need to skim off the scum, both ways will help you achieve a clear looking broth.

5. When the ox tail meat is tender and falling from the bone, scoop them out and remove the meat and reserve it for having with your broth later. Return the bones to the pot if you are using a slow cooker or stove top.

6. In the final couple of hours of cooking add in your vegetables and herbs, if using a slow cooker or stove top.Once the desired cooking time has been reached use a large slotted spoon or tong to remove the bones and veggies.

7. Using a large bowl and fine mesh strainer lined with a muslin cloth, strain the liquid, rinsing out the cloth and sieve of any sediments as you go.

8. Taste for salt and adjust if necessary.

9. Pour into desired container/s and refrigerate, when the fat has solidified on top scoop it off for later use.

10. Portion it up how you like and serve with any meat you reserved from earlier in the cooking process, sip the broth on its own, or add to your soups and stews etc.

CHICKEN BONE BROTH

Preparation time: 10 mins

Cooking time: 4 - 6 hrs

Ingredients: Yields approx 2-3 litres using an 8 litre pot

- 1 onion roughly chopped
- 1 leek roughly chopped including green leaves
- 2 carrots roughly chopped
- 2 stalks of celery roughly chopped including leaves
- 2kgs (4lb) raw or cooked chicken bones (carcass/frames, wings and wing tips,legs/drumsticks)

- 2 bay leaves
- Small bunch of herbs e.g. parsley, thyme, rosemary
- Pink salt

Method:

1. Preheat your oven to 200 degrees, and liberally salt the bones. Roast for around 30-40 mins till well browned. You can also roast your veggies at the same time if you want; just set them aside after roasting if you are using a slow cooker or stove top method.

2. Put the bones into the pot that you are using and pour some boiling water into the roasting tray. Allow it to stand for few minutes. Using a spatula, scrape up any of the caramelised bits on the bottom of the pan and add this to the pot.

3. If you are using a pressure cooker or instant pot, add the remainder of ingredients to the pot and top up with water. Cook for manufactures recommended length of time.

4. If using a slow cooker or stove top method, add in the apple cider vinegar and top up with water and simmer for preferred amount of time. For stove top method bring the bones to a boil then scoop off any scum/foam that appears on the surface then reduce heat to a simmer. If you just simmer the bones and don't boil them first you won't need to skim off the scum, both ways will help you achieve a clear looking broth.having with your broth later.

5. When the drumstick meat is tender and falling from the bone, scoop them out and remove the meat and reserve it for having with your broth later. Return the bones to the pot if you are using a slow cooker or stove top.

6. In the final couple of hours of cooking add in your vegetables and herbs, if using a slow cooker or stove top.

7. Once the desired cooking time has been reached use a large slotted spoon or tong to remove the bones and veggies.

8. Using a large bowl and fine mesh strainer lined with a muslin cloth strain the liquid, rinsing out the cloth and sieve of any sediments as you go.

9. Taste for salt and adjust if necessary.

10. Pour into desired container/s and refrigerate, when the fat has solidified on top scoop it off for later use.

11. Portion it up how you like and serve with any meat you reserved from earlier in the cooking process, sip on its own or add to your soups and stews etc.

FISH BONE BROTH

	Preparation time: 10 mins		Cooking time: 4-6 hours		Total time: 1 hour 45 minutes

It is very important to use fish bones from non oily fish such as snapper, cod or flounder, to avoid a stock that tastes too fishy. Fish frames including the very gelatinous heads are easily sourced for very little money from your local fish markets. I like to sweat my fish bones over a gentle heat, being mindful of them catching as they can burn easily. This helps bring out the flavour of the bones rather than roasting them. This style of broth I prefer to make on the stove top.

Ingredients: Yields approximately 2 litres using a 6 litre pot

- 2 kg (4 ½ lb) raw fish bones (see note above)
- 2-3 tbsp olive oil
- 1 leek chopped
- 1 onion chopped

- Small bunch of herbs for example dill, tarragon, parsley
- 2-3 bay leaves
- 3 litres of filtered water

Method:

1. Wash the bones in plenty of cold water. Discard any bloody bits near the heads. Gently warm the olive oil in a large stock pot or large saucepan. Add the bones and stir until you can smell cooked fish rather than raw fish. The bones should not brown.

2. Add all the remaining ingredients and bring to the boil. Skim away any white foam that appears. Simmer gently, uncovered, for 1 ½ hours then strain through a fine meshed sieve lined with a muslin cloth.

3. There will be little to no fat that will form on the top of the stock. Pour into jars and refrigerate; use within 5 days or freeze.

CAESAR DRESSING

Preparation time:
10 mins

Total time:
10 minutes

Ingredients:

- 125g (½ cup) coconut cream
- 200g (2/3 cup) avocado oil
- 30g (1 tbsp) olive oil

- 60g (2 tbsp) lemon juice
- Salt
- 2 cloves garlic

Method:

1. Place all ingredients in an up-right blender and blend until combined

2. Store in an airtight container and chill.

3. If you use the dressing at a later stage and it has separated, shake the container firmly to get the right consistency again.

COCONUT BUTTER

Preparation time: 05 mins	Cooking time: 10 mins	Total time: 15 mins

Coconut butter is a great spread that can be used in many different ways. Use it as a butter substitute, add a spoonful to smoothies or use it to make AIP mayo.

Ingredients:

- 500g (2 cups) coconut flakes
- 60ml (2 tbsp) coconut oil

Method:

TIP - The key to making coconut butter is to get the right consistency, which depends on the climate you live in and the fat contents of the coconut flakes.Making coconut butter takes some time. A bigger batch is therefore a good idea.

Store it in the fridge in an airtight container, it keeps for weeks, or freeze some for later use. It's essential to have a high powered blender or food processor to break the coconut down enough to form a paste.

1. Place the coconut flakes in a food processor and run the machine until you get a smooth buttery texture, this will take somewhere between 3 to 10 minutes.

2. Allow the machine to rest a little in between, so the whole mixture doesn't get too hot.

3. If the flakes do not get buttery add the coconut oil, a little at a time

4. The speed of the food processor will make the mixture hot and it may not look like butter. Not to worry, just allow cooling and it will return to the right consistency.

How easy a recipe is that?

Nutritional values are manually calculated and based on the ingredients specified.

Nutritional value per serving: Calories: 3073.3 Fat: 240.0g. Saturated Fat: 213.9g. Sodium: 1332.0mg. Carbohydrate 234.0g Protein: 13.0g. Dietary fibre: 13.0g

COCONUT YOGHURT

Preparation time: 05 mins

Cooking time: 10 mins

Total time: 10 mins plus cooling & 8-12 hrs culturing time

There is nothing like thick creamy coconut yogurt, however the store bought varieties are quite expensive. It's quite easy and inexpensive to make your own at home. There are so many homemade coconut yoghurt recipes around; this is a recipe I have created after trying quite a few different methods and it delivers a lovely thick, creamy, tangy yoghurt every time.Many commercial coconut yoghurts use tapioca starch as a thickener and stabiliser to prevent separation, and I have adopted the same theory with my recipe.

This recipe is very quick to prepare, the hard part is waiting for it to culture then to chill in the fridge. However it is well worth the wait. It is so adaptable and can be utilised in so many different ways.

Ingredients:

- Makes 800ml (27 fl.oz)

- 800ml coconut cream

- 1 tbsp tapioca starch

- 1-2 tsp grass fed gelatine granules

- 1-2 tsp pure maple syrup or raw honey (optional)

- Pinch of pink salt

- 2-3 pro-biotic capsules

Method:

1. Pour ¼ cup of coconut cream into a small dish and mix in the tapioca starch until there are no lumps.

2. Pour the remaining coconut cream, the tapioca starch mixture and the rest of the ingredients, except for the probiotics, in to a small saucepan.

3. Bring the mixture to a medium heat, continually stirring. Once it has reached a medium heat continue to stir for another couple of minutes; ensuring the gelatine has dissolved.

4. Take off the heat and allow cooling completely until it is room temperature.

5. Once it has cooled to room temperature empty the probiotic capsules into the mixture and stir to combine. They may form little lumps, this is fine, they will dissolve while the yogurt is culturing.

6. Pour the yoghurt mixture into a yogurt maker and culture for up to 12 hrs. The longer you allow it to culture, the tangier it will taste.

7. Once it has cultured, give it a little shake if any separation has occurred, and put in the fridge to chill.

SWEET POTATO FRIES

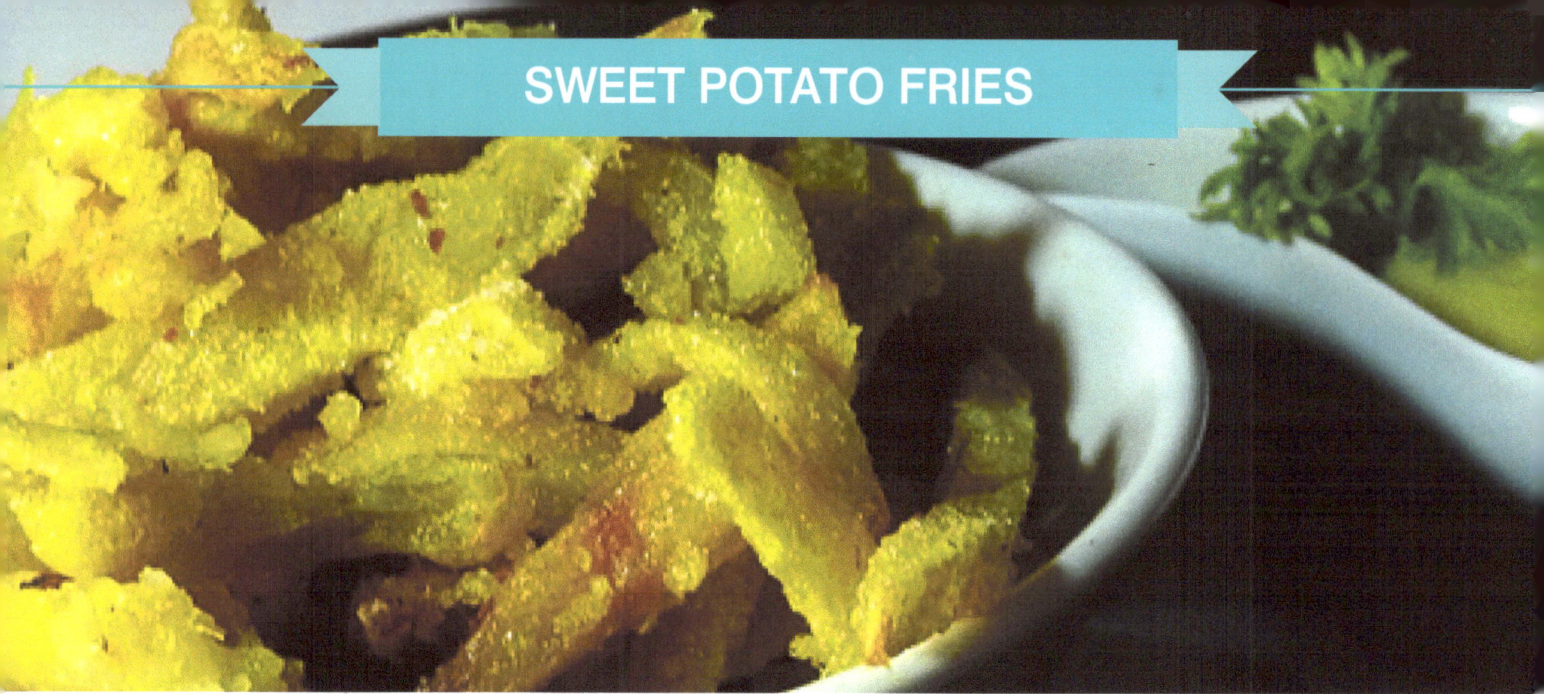

Preparation time: 10 mins

Cooking time: 10 mins

Total time: 20 mins

Everyone loves fries and just because you are on AIP doesn't mean you have to miss out!! If you can get some duck fat to fry these babies the flavour is spectacular!

Ingredients:

Serves 4

- 4 large sweet potatoes (peeled and cut into thin strips)
- 90gr (3 tbsp) tapioca starch
- Ice cold water
- 250gr (1 cup) Coyo yoghurt
- 10gr (1 tsp) chopped mint leaves
- 60gr (2 tbsp) peeled, de-seeded cucumber, cut in small cubes

- 60ml (2 tbsp) coconut oil
- Oil or fat of choice for frying
- Pink salt
- 30g (1tbsp) dried herbs e.g. ground turmeric, oregano, thyme, sage, rosemary or your favourite combination of these

Method:

1. Pre- heat your deep fryer to 140 degrees (284 F).
2. Ensure the fries are about 1 cm (½ inch) square.
3. Fry them in the oil for 4 minutes, drain on kitchen paper.
4. While the fries are draining, but still hot, sprinkle the herbs and salt over them and shake through.
5. Meanwhile make the dip by combining the yoghurt with the mint and cucumber, season with a little salt.
6. Increase the heat of the fryer to 180 degrees (325 F)
7. Mix the tapioca starch with the cold water and combine to a batter.
8. Dip the fries in small batches in the batter to avoid sticking, and finish for 2 minutes until golden and crisp.
9. Serve with a dip made from the Coyo, mint and cucumber.

Nutritional values are manually calculated and based on the ingredients specified.
Nutritional value per serving: Calories: 352.7. Fat: 25.4 g Saturated Fat: 1.9 g. Sodium: 16.9 mg. Sugar: 0.0 g Carbohydrate 35.1 g. Protein: 3.5 g. Dietary fibre: 3.9 g

MAYONNAISE

Classic French cuisine identifies five mother sauces. All of these are hot sauces, but as mayonnaise is a cold sauce it is not one of them. Mayonnaise has been so prominently positioned in the culinary world today and has all the characteristics of a mother sauce. In my opinion it should be added to the list of five.

Having a good mayonnaise that suits the AIP lifestyle is versatile so can be used for many dishes.

The process of making a dressing taught us that oil and acidity (vinegar or lemon juice) do not mix very well, and to make a solid cold sauce we need an aid or substitute. Especially as we are not using eggs or mustard.

Coconut butter becomes our aid to make delicious AIP mayonnaise.

Ingredients:

* 125g (½ cup) coconut butter

* 125ml (½ cup) warm filtered water

* 60ml (¼ cup) olive oil

* 2 cloves garlic

* 90ml (3tbsp) lemon juice

* 60gr (2 tbsp) peeled, de-seeded cucumber, cut in small cubes

* 2-3 pro-biotic capsules

Method:

1. Place all ingredients in a food processor and blend to combine into a smooth texture.

2. Allow cooling for 10 minutes before use.

Store in an airtight container, it will last for weeks when chilled

YOGHURT DRESSING

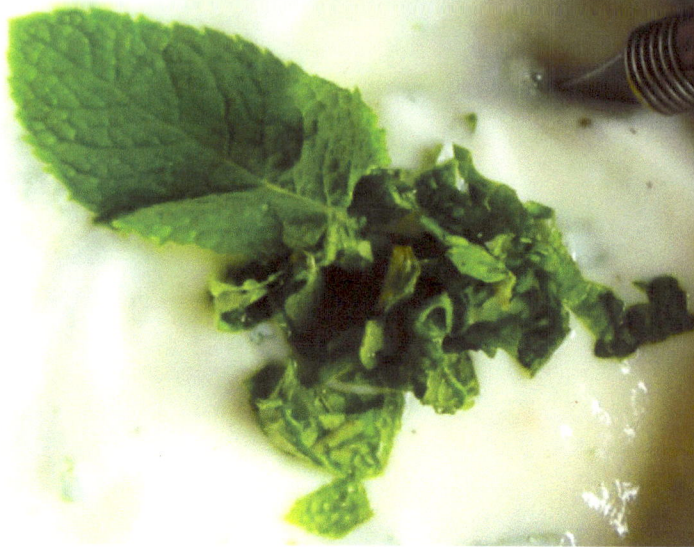

Ingredients:

- 125g (½ cup) coconut yoghurt (Coyo)
- ½ avocado (cut in small pieces)
- 30g (1 tbsp) olive oil
- 60ml (2 tbsp) lemon juice
- 1g (1 tsp) raw honey
- 1 clove garlic
- 30g (¼ cup) chopped fresh dill
- Sea salt
- 60ml (¼ cup) filtered water

Method:

1. Place all ingredients in an up-right blender and blend to combine into a smooth texture.
2. Store in an airtight container and chill.

ZUCCHINI CHEESE

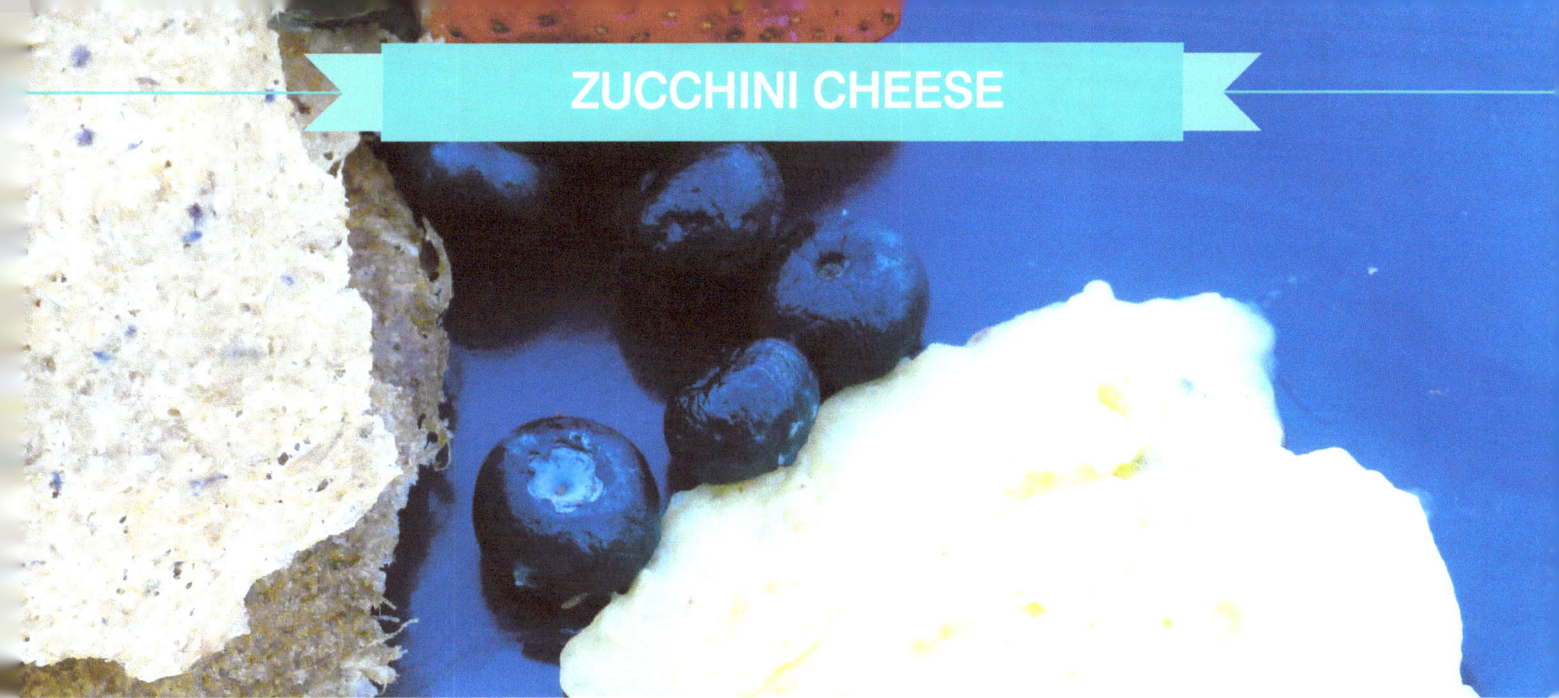

Preparation time: 25 minutes

Cooking time: 0 minutes

Chilling / Cooling Time: 2 hrs

Total time: 2 hrs 25 min

No need to be sad about giving up cheese, who would have thought you could get the same flavour and texture from zucchini? You can easily add some of your favourite herbs to this or even a pinch or two of ground turmeric, for extra anti-inflammatory benefits and a hint of yellow colour. This works well chopped up, grated into salads or as a side.

Ingredients: Serves 4

- 250g (1 cup) zucchini (peeled and cut small)
- 60ml (¼ cup) water
- 45g (1 ½ tbsp.) grass fed gelatine granules
- 30ml (1 tbsp) olive oil
- Pink salt
- 15ml (1tsp) lemon juice

Method:

1. Place the zucchini with the water in a small sauce pan and bring to a slow boil, simmer until softened, about 10 to 12 minutes.

2. Drain the water out and transfer to a blender, add the oil, salt and lemon juice, and blend until smooth.
3. Return the mix to the sauce pan, add the gelatin and heat until it boils again.
4. Transfer the mix to a mould or rimmed tray and allow cooling for 2 hours in the fridge.
5. Slice in desired pieces and serve with vegetable crackers.

Nutritional values are manually calculated and based on the ingredients specified.
Nutritional value per serving: Calories: 291.4. Fat: 13.7g Saturated Fat: 1.8g Sodium: 147.0mg. Sugar: 2.1g Carbohydrate 4.1g Protein: 39.5g Dietary fibre: 1.4g

SOUPS

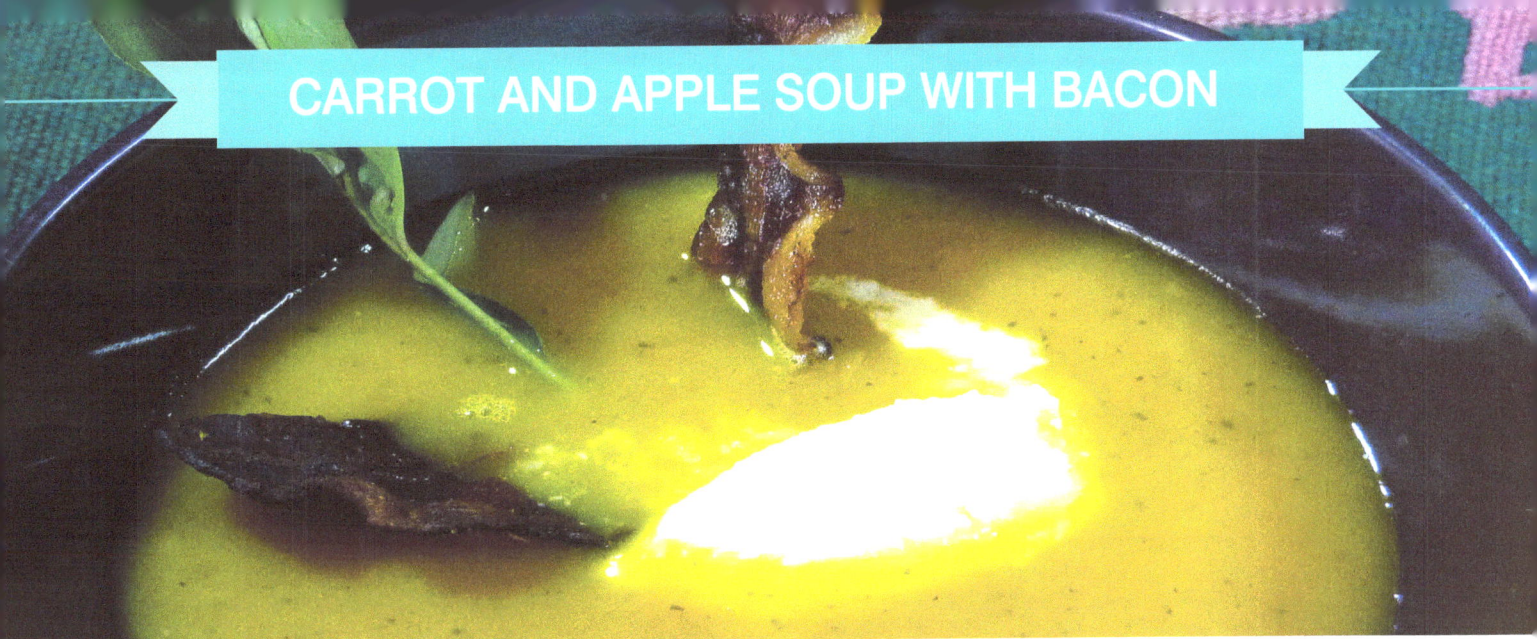

CARROT AND APPLE SOUP WITH BACON

Preparation time: 15 mins

Cooking time: 20 mins

Total time: 35 mins

Carrot and apple combine well in this carotene rich concoction. I have added a little orange juice for a sour touch and some smoky bacon to make it unique. Vietnamese coriander is known to clean the blood and adds another flavour dimension. If you can find it great, if not, use normal coriander leaves. In the recipe I boil the veggies, if you have a little extra time oven roast them for a more intense flavour. Roast two of the apples and add in one fresh when you blend the soup. Either way it's a flavoursome soup!!

For a spicy kick you can roast a half inch piece of ginger and turmeric and peel before blending. This will also have an anti-inflammatory effect on the body.

Ingredients: Serves 4

- 1 litre (4 cups) chicken broth
- 3 medium sized apples (cut small) I prefer granny smith
- 1 small onion (cut in pieces)
- 3 cloves of garlic
- 125ml (½ cup) orange juice
- 4 rashes of bacon   • Sea salt
- 30gr (3 tbsp) Vietnamese coriander
- 60ml (4 tbsp) coconut cream

Method:

1. Place the carrots and apples (I don't peel them to catch all of the nutrients) with the onion, orange juice, coriander and the bacon in a stockpot. Add the chicken stock and bring to a boil.
2. Lower the heat and simmer for 20 minutes.
3. Remove the bacon from the pot and keep aside.
4. Transfer (with the use of a slotted spoon) the solids from the pot to an up-right blender, add a little stock and blend until smooth.
5. Return the blended solids to the pot and strain through a sieve.
6. Check for taste and keep warm.
7. Fry the bacon rashes until crisp.
8. Serve the soup piping hot with a gentle dollop of coconut cream, add the bacon.

Nutritional values are manually calculated and based on the ingredients specified.
Nutritional value per serving: Calories: 223.9 Fat: 5.5g Saturated Fat: 1.7g. Sodium: 791.4mg. Sugar: 16.0g Carbohydrate 30.4g Protein: 13.5g Dietary fibre: 4.5g

CELERY SOUP WITH CRISPY CHICKEN SKIN

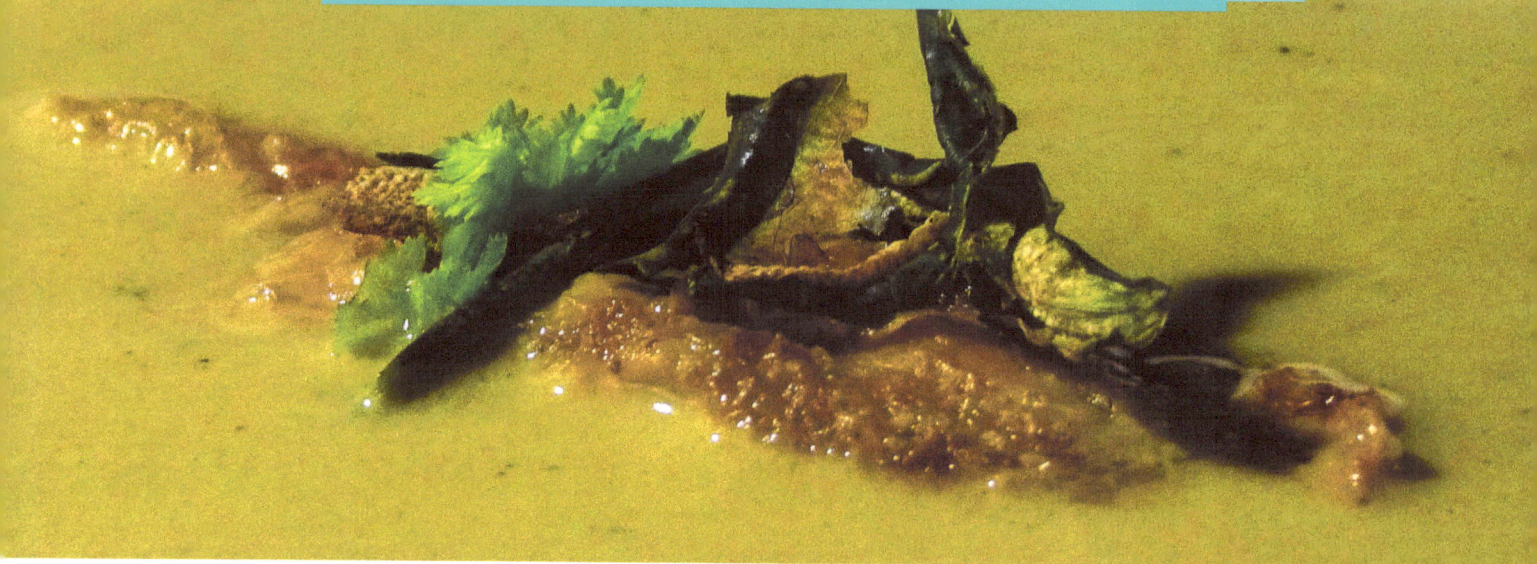

Preparation time: 15 mins

Cooking time: 20 mins

Total time: 35 mins

Celery is a vegetable often regarded as an "add in". We add it to stocks, braised meats and chop some for some crunch in a salad. Celery is however a star in its own right packed full of anti-inflammatory properties. Celery is rich in vitamin K, foliate and fibre, and most of all it is delicious. This recipe is crunchy and so tasty! Who doesn't love crispy chicken skin!?

Ingredients: Serves 4

- 1 litre (4 cups) chicken broth
- 1 medium sized onion (cut small)
- 30gr (2 tbsp) coriander stems and leaves
- Skin of half a cucumber
- 60 ml (2 tbsp) olive oil

- 500gr (2 cups) celery (roughly chopped)
- 2 cloves garlic (crushed)
- 4 pieces chicken skin
- 125 ml (½ cup) coconut cream
- Pink salt

Method:

1. Pre-heat an oven to 160 degrees (320 F).
2. Place the cucumber skin and the chicken skin on a baking tray, sprinkle with salt and roast until crisp in the oven, this takes about 20 minutes.
3. Meanwhile heat the oil in a stockpot, add the onion, garlic, coriander and celery to the pan and fry for two minutes.
4. Add the broth and bring to a boil, lower the heat and simmer for 15 minutes.
5. Add the coconut, bring back to the boil and transfer to an up-right blender. Blend smooth and press the soup through a sieve. Check for taste.
6. Divide the soup over serving bowls and top with the chicken skin and cucumber crisps.
7. Serve piping hot.

Nutritional values are manually calculated and based on the ingredients specified.
Nutritional value per serving: Calories: 147.4 Fat: 9.1g Saturated Fat: 2.7g. Sodium: 1090.0 mg. Sugar: 1.6g Carbohydrate 8.3g Protein: 9.5g Dietary fibre: 2.5 g

CHINESE MUSHROOM SOUP

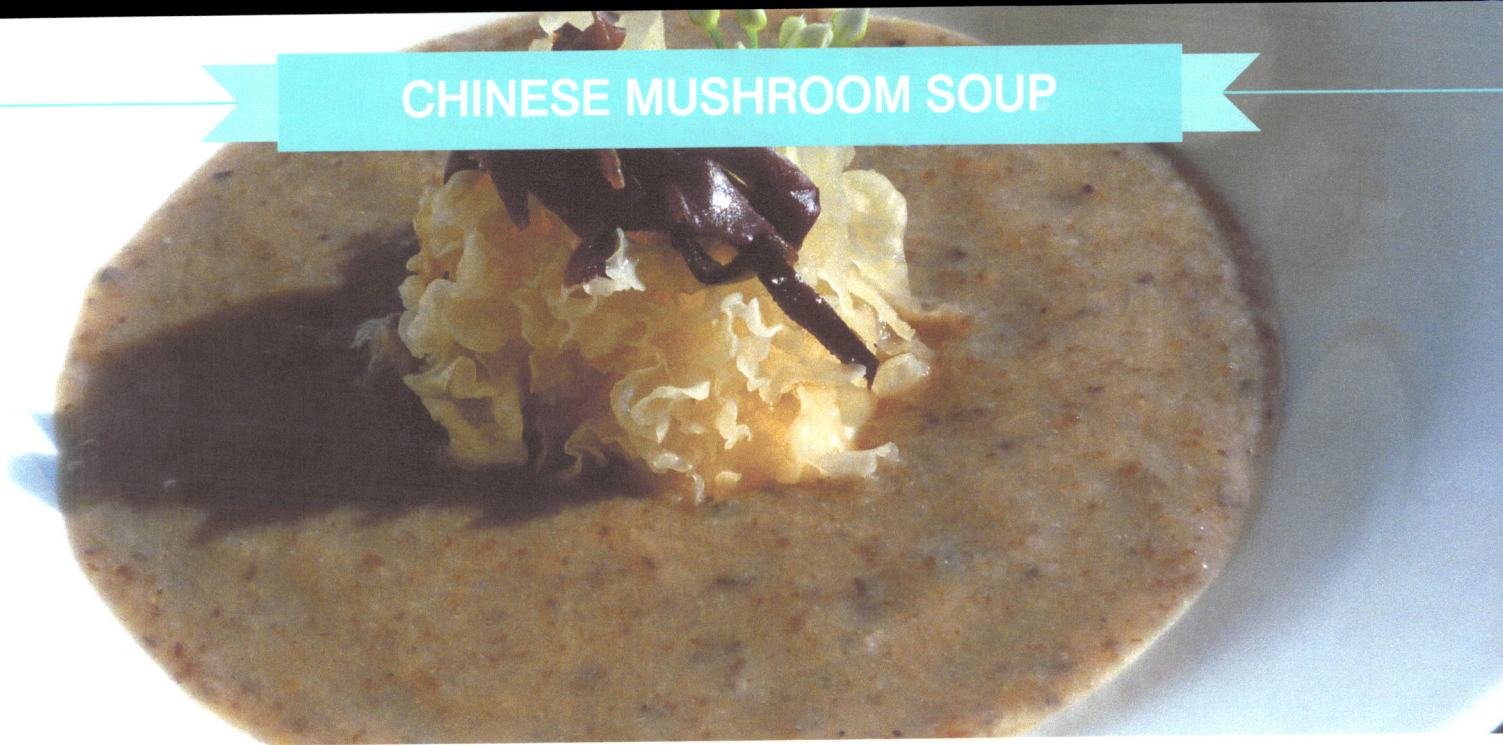

Preparation time: 02 hrs

Cooking time: 10 mins

Total time: 02 hrs 10 mins

Chinese mushrooms have been known for their medicinal health benefits for at least 6000 years. Shi-Take, or black Chinese mushrooms, are the most well known and the most available too. If you do come across some other varieties like wood ear or white fungus in dried form, bring some home. In dried form they last forever, and when turned into a soup with their soaking water and/or a strong bone broth, you create a very nourishing, flavourful and delicious soup. The health benefits are unprecedented, from cell binding of blood vessels, to richness in iron. Super easy and quick to make, this recipe will please everyone's palate.

Ingredients: Serves 4

- 1 litre (4 cups) bone broth or 2/3 bone broth and 1/3 soaking water

- 50gr (1 ½ oz) dried wood ear fungus

- Pink salt

- 200gr (6 ½ oz) black dried Chinese Shi-Take mushrooms

- 50gr (1 ½ oz) dried white fungus

Method:

1. Soak the dried mushrooms in double the amount of water as the mushrooms, especially the wood ear; they will become about 3 times their dried size.

2. Add the soaked mushrooms to a stockpot with some soaking water and the bone broth, the ratio is your preference.
3. Bring to a boil, lower the heat and simmer for 15 minutes.
4. Transfer the mix to an up-right blender and blend until very smooth.
5. Check for taste and serve with some chopped mushrooms.

Nutritional values are manually calculated and based on the ingredients specified.
Nutritional value per serving: Calories: 323.0. Fat: 12.8g Saturated Fat: 4.3g. Sodium: 245.8mg Sugar: 2.9g Carbohydrate 54.1g Protein: 23.3g Dietary fibre: 2.4g

NAN'S CHICKEN SOUP

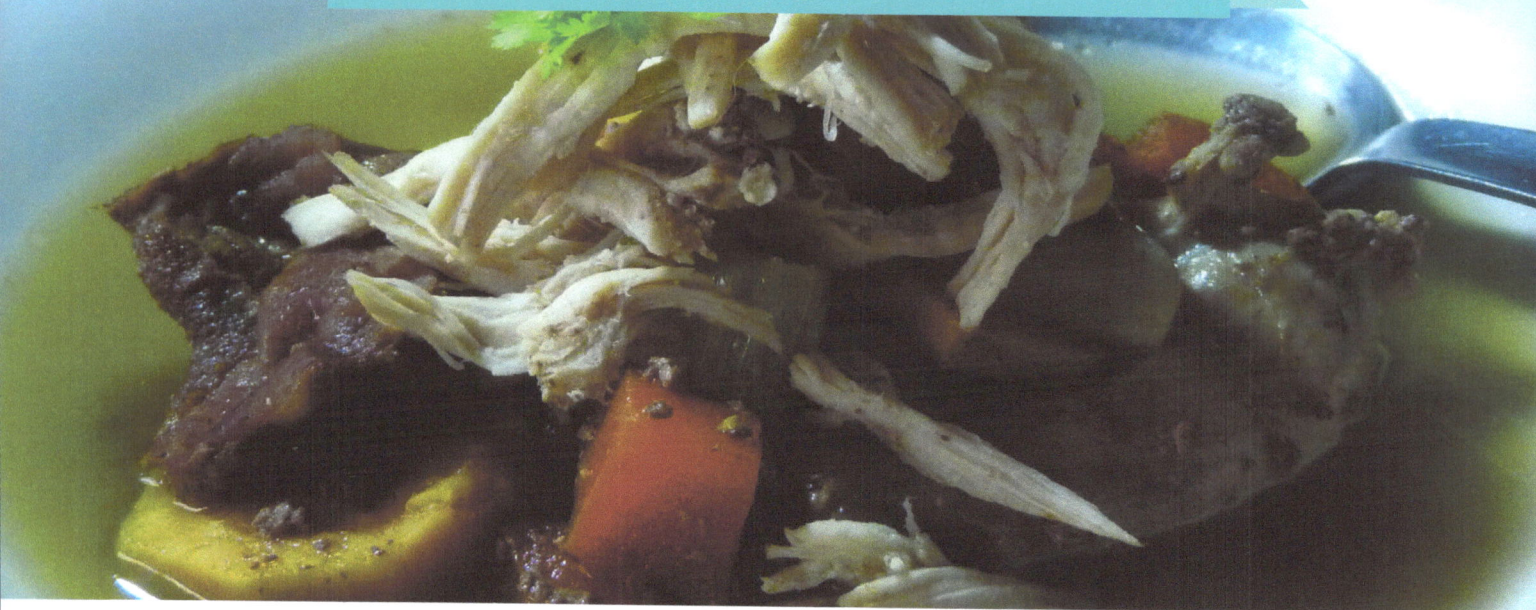

Preparation time:
15 mins

Cooking time:
30 mins

Total time:
55 mins

Have you ever tried essence of chicken? This strong chicken broth is known for many medicinal properties and is a trusted remedy for many illnesses. It is made by crushing whole chickens and steaming them for 12 hours in a covered pot on a wood fired steamer. The extracted juice is called essence of chicken. You will find it in good delicatessens or specialty food emporiums.

This procedure is surely not an option for all, but you can buy some and add it to this chicken soup recipe. Already full of goodies some essence of chicken will make it even more rich and nutritious.

Ingredients: Serves 4

- 1 litre (4 cups) chicken broth (or 750 ml (3 cups) broth and 250 ml (1 cup) essence of chicken

- 125gr (½ cup) celery   • 4 pieces chicken neck

- 1 medium onion   • Pink salt

- 125gr (½ cup) turnips

- 180gr (6 oz) chicken breast

- 60gr (2 tbsp) parsley or coriander stems

- 125gr (½ cup) sweet potato

- 125gr (½ cup) carrots

- 8 pieces chicken gizzard

Method:

1. Place all ingredients in a stockpot and bring to a boil, lower the heat and simmer for 30 minutes.
2. Strain the stock through a cheese cloth and return the other ingredients, except for the chicken breast, to the sieved broth. Simmer the veggies until tender.
3. Shred the chicken breast by hand.
4. Check the soup for taste and divide over bowls.
5. Top with the shredded chicken and garnish with coriander leaves.
6. Serve piping hot.

Nutritional values are manually calculated and based on the ingredients specified.
Nutritional value per serving: Calories: 221.5 Fat: 4.8g Saturated Fat: 1.2g. Sodium: 463.9mg. Sugar: 9.5g Carbohydrate 21.9g Protein: 21.9g Dietary fibre: 3.9g

PUMPKIN AND PEAR SOUP WITH BACON BITS

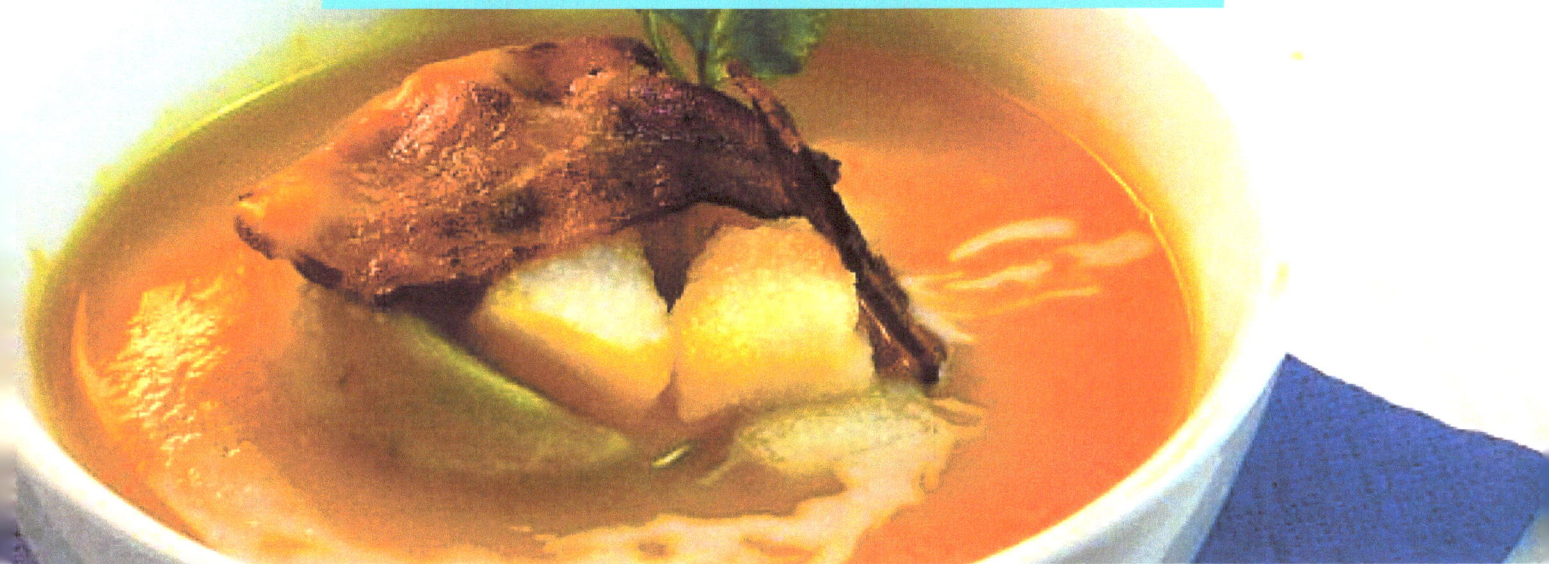

Preparation time: 10 mins

Cooking time: 20 mins

Total time: 30 mins

The sweet flavours of fruit pair superbly with savoury dishes, as proven in this recipe. The sweet juices of the pears provide a palate satisfying tang, added to the pumpkin and the thyme. Smoky and crisp bacon bits give it another textural dimension, and the salty smoky taste is simple yet divine!

Ingredients:
Serves 4

- 30 ml (1 tbsp) olive oil
- 250ml (1 cup) coconut milk
- 500g (2 cups) pumpkin or butternut squash
- 350g (1 ½ cup) leeks (cut small)
- 3 pears (peeled, cored and cut small)

- 1 litre (4 cups) bone broth (homemade if possible)
- 8 rashes smoked bacon
- Pink salt
- 250g (1 cup) onion (chopped)
- 10g (1 tsp) chopped fresh thyme

Method:

1. Heat the oil in a stock pot on medium heat, add the leeks and cook for 5 minutes.
2. Add the onions, mix well. Add the pumpkin, pears and thyme and the vegetable stock, bring to a soft boil. Lower the heat and cook for another 15 minutes.
3. Transfer the solids to an up-right blender, add some of the liquid and blend smooth.
4. Return the mix back to the stock pot and stir in the coconut milk.
   While the soup is cooking, fry the bacon rashes in a skillet until crisp, 2 to 3 minutes, drain on kitchen paper and allow cooling.
5. Re-heat the soup to boiling point and season with salt.
6. Break the bacon into small pieces over the soup and serve hot.

Nutritional values are manually calculated and based on the ingredients specified.
Nutritional value per serving: Calories: 162.9. Fat: 2.8g. Saturated Fat: 1.5g. Sodium: 152.8mg. Carbohydrate 34.0g Protein: 2.8g. Dietary fibre: 8.7g.

SEAFOOD CHOWDER

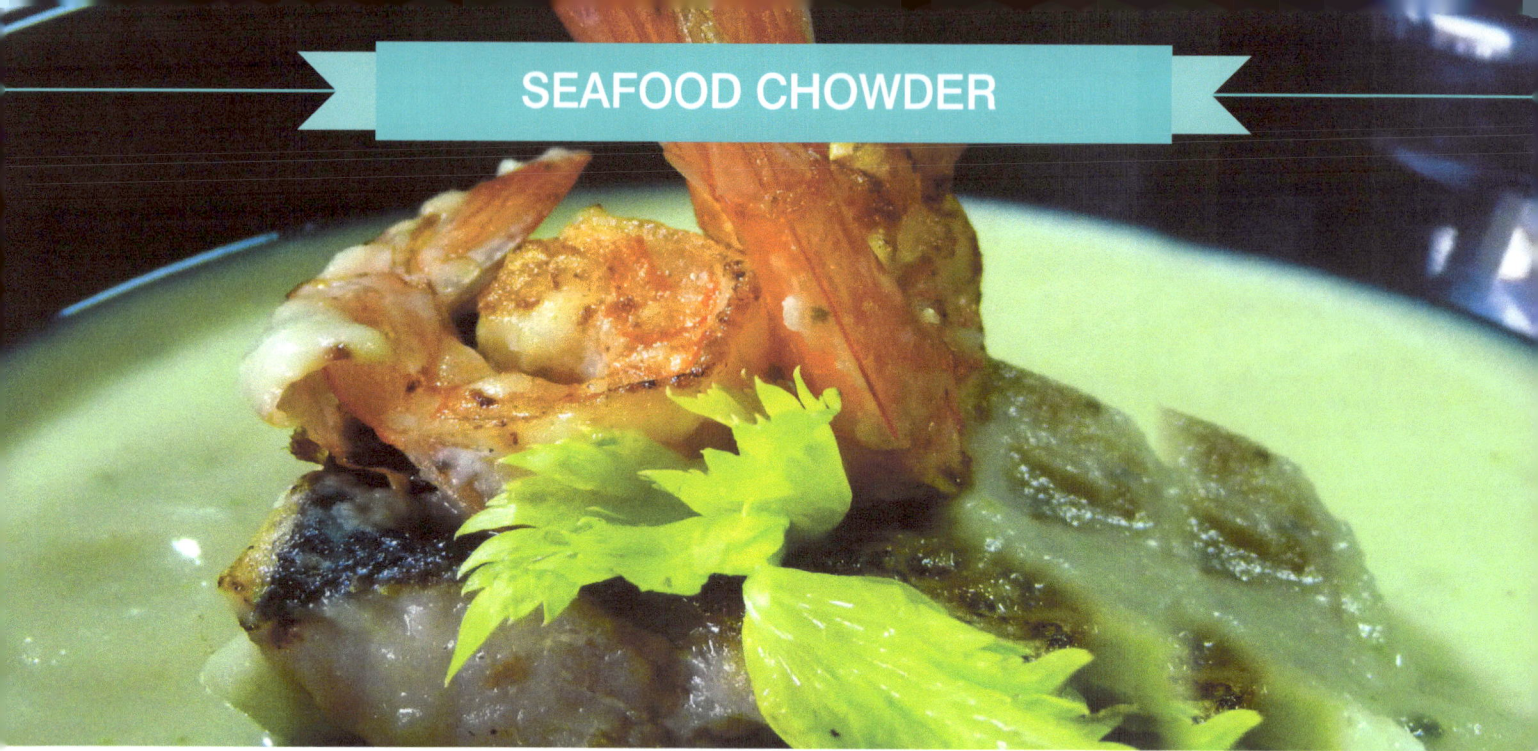

Preparation time: 15 mins	Cooking time: 20 mins	Total time: 35 mins

Chowder was a firm favourite pre-AIP; however it's traditionally full of corn and cream, and often nightshades. I replaced the cream in this hearty seafood soup with vegetables that provide the perfect creaminess you'll be looking for in chowder.

Ingredients: Serves 4

- 30 ml (1 tbsp) olive oil
- A few coriander stalks
- 250gr (1 cup) turnips (cut small)
- 125 ml (½ cup) coconut milk
- 8 medium sized prawns (divined, tail on)

- 1 litre (4 cups) seafood broth
- Pink salt
- 4 pieces black cod (90gr, 3 oz, each)
- 250gr (1 cup) cauliflower (cut small)

Method:

1. Bring the seafood broth with the cauliflower, turnips and coriander stalks to a boil, lower the heat and simmer until soft, about 15 minutes.

2. Meanwhile heat the olive oil to medium heat in a skillet and fry the cod and prawns for 1 to 2 minutes, until cooked. Remove from the pan and drain on kitchen paper.

3. When the vegetables in the broth are soft and have cooled, transfer to an up-right blender and blend smooth. Return to the pan and season.

4. Ladle the chowder into bowls; add a piece of cod to each bowl, followed by 2 prawns.

5. Serve the chowder piping hot.

Nutritional values are manually calculated and based on the ingredients specified.
Nutritional value per serving: Calories: 455.7 Fat: 13.9g Saturated Fat: 0.7g Sodium: 2615.4mg. Sugar: 6.0g Carbohydrate 33.4g Protein: 44.5g Dietary fibre: 2.5g

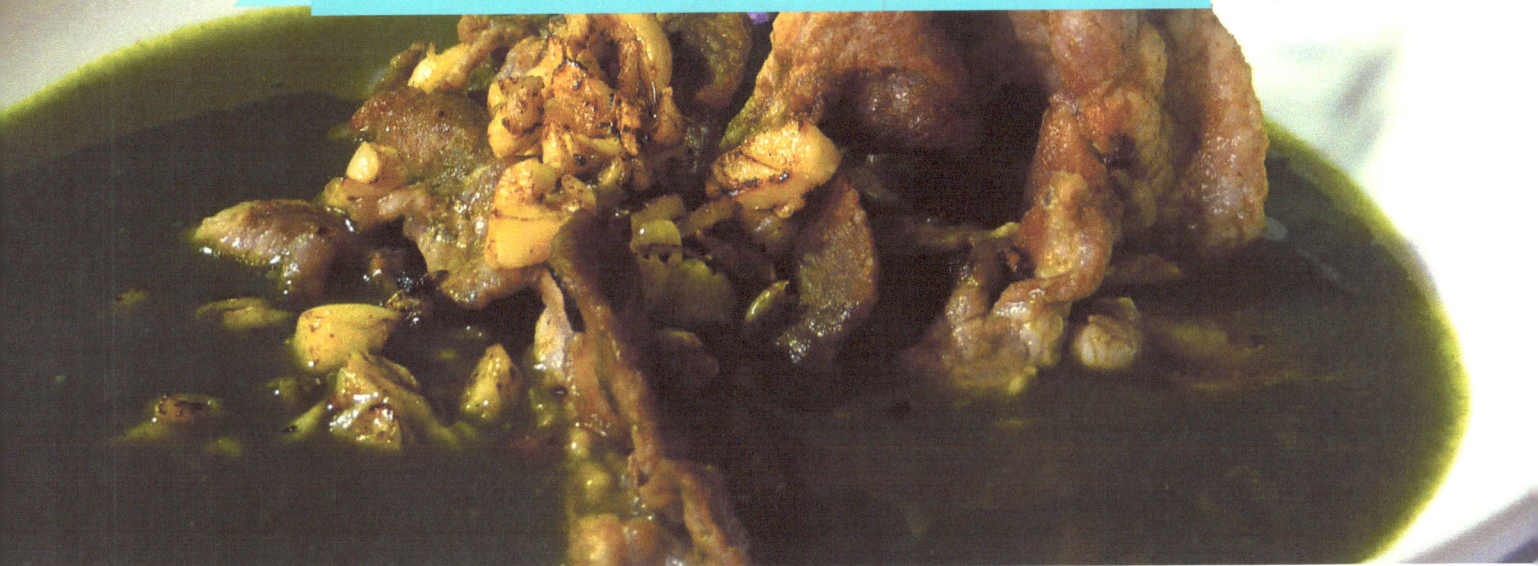

WATERCRESS SOUP WITH FRIED LAMB LEG AND ROASTED GARLIC

Preparation time: 15 mins

Cooking time: 20 mins

Total time: 35 mins

Leafy greens are very important in your diet while following AIP. They provide lots of nutrients and lovely colours. Watercress is one of them, which I combined here with thinly sliced lamb leg and pungent roasted garlic for some punch. Another quick easy mid-week sensation!

Ingredients:
Serves 4

- 1 litre (4 cups) bone broth
- 1 medium sized onion (cut in pieces)
- 4 thin slices lamb leg steaks
- 500gr (2 cups) watercress (roughly chopped)

- 2 cloves garlic (crushed)
- 2 cloves garlic (crushed)
- 60 ml (2 tbsp) olive oil • Pink salt
- 90gr (3 tbsp) chopped garlic

Method:

1. Place the watercress with the broth, onion and garlic in a stockpot.
2. Bring to a boil, lower the heat and simmer for 15 minutes.
3. Transfer to an up-right blender and blend smooth.
4. Return to the pot and check for taste.
5. Heat the oil in a skillet to high heat and fry the lamb leg for 2 minutes. Remove from the pan and set the heat to medium.
6. Add the chopped garlic and fry, while continuously stirring, until the garlic is golden brown and fragrant. Usually for 1-2 minutes.
7. Place a slice of the lamb leg in a soup bowl or plate, top with the soup and sprinkle some roasted garlic over the meat.
8. Serve piping hot.

Nutritional values are manually calculated and based on the ingredients specified.
Nutritional value per serving: Calories: 413.8 Fat: 16.6g Saturated Fat: 5.8g Sodium: 354.0mg. Sugar: 1.6g Carbohydrate 27.7g Protein: 40.5g Dietary fibre: 2.2g

SALADS

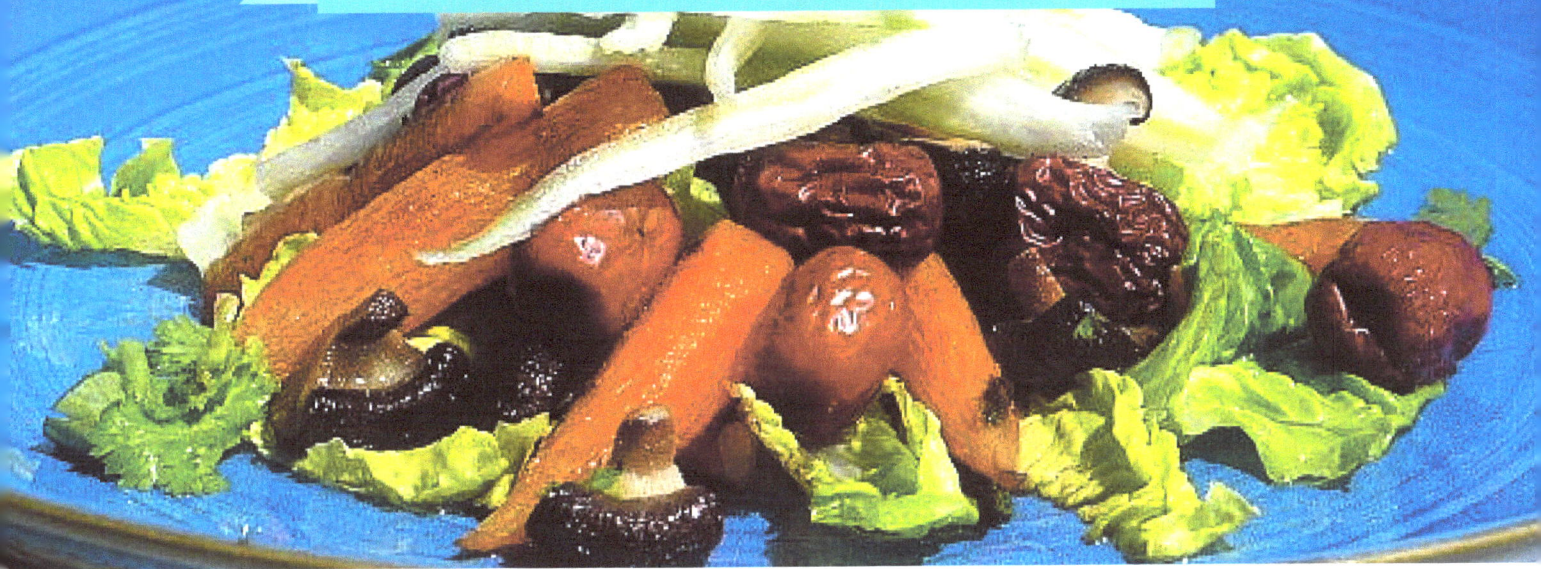

BABY CARROT, DATE AND MUSHROOM SALAD WITH CRUNCHY CELERY

Preparation time: 15 mins

Cooking time: 05 mins

Total time: 20 mins

Dates are a fantastic fruit for salads and desserts, and are a good source of dietary potassium. I prefer fresh medjool dates however the dried varieties work just as well. This salad will make a lovely lunch dish with added flavour from the lightly fried mushrooms. Crunchiness from the celery gives a nice touch to this light summer meal.

Ingredients:

Serves 4

- 250g (1 cup) baby carrots (cut lengthwise in quarters)

- 16 fresh dates or 4 oz dried dates (I love medjool dates!)

- 90g (3 tbsp) fresh orange juice

- 30g (2 tbsp) chopped coriander leaves

- 2 large celery stalks (sliced in 2 ½ inch strips)

- 30ml (1 tbsp) olive oil   • 90ml (3 tbsp) lemon juice

- 120ml (4 tbsp) olive oil   • Pink salt

- 375g (1 ½ cup) brown bottom mushrooms (quartered)

Method:

1. Heat 1 tbsp of olive oil in a frying pan on medium heat. Add the mushrooms and fry for 2 minutes.
2. Combine the orange, lemon juice, and the remaining olive oil and palm sugar in a mixing bowl.
3. Add the baby carrots and the mushrooms and mix. Allow resting for 5 minutes.
4. When you use fresh dates do not add them to the dressing. If you use dried dates cut them in 3 or 4 equal pieces and add to the dressing. Mix well.
5. Place the salad on 4 individual plates and top with the celery strips.
6. When you use fresh dates, arrange them around the salad.

Nutritional values are manually calculated and based on the ingredients specified.
Nutritional value per serving: Calories: 171.1 Fat: 3.9g. Saturated Fat: 0.5g. Sodium: 72.0mg Carbohydrate 35.1g Protein: 3.3g. Dietary fibre: 5.3g.

BEETROOT CARPACCIO WITH CRAB SALAD AND AVOCADO

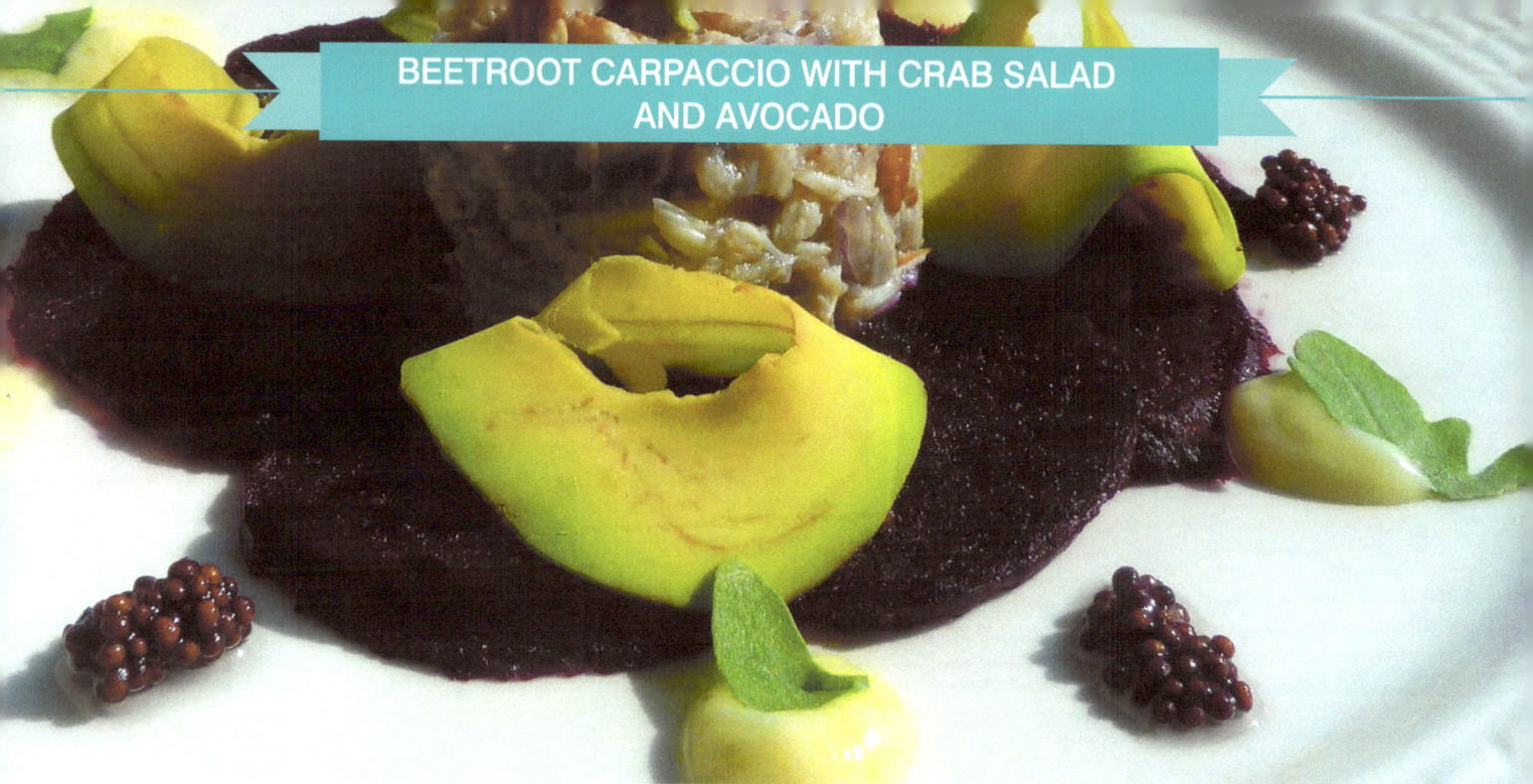

Preparation time: 35 mins

Cooking time: 15 mins

Total time: 50 mins

This dish has colourful healthy ingredients like beetroot, which is low in fat, full of vitamins and minerals and loaded with antioxidants. The avocados are high in healthy fats and also loaded with vitamins, 20 different ones to be precise! Paired with sweet crab this combination can hardly go wrong. Perfect summer salad!! Prawns would also be perfect in this dish.

Ingredients: Serves 4

- 450gr (1 pound crabmeat)
- 1 small red onion (finely sliced)
- 90gr (3 tbsp) coconut mayonnaise
- Sea salt

- 1 small red onion (finely sliced)
- 2 medium sized avocados (peeled, de-seeded and sliced lengthwise)
- 60gr (2 tbsp) salmon caviar

Method:

1. Combine the crabmeat with the onion and season with a little salt.
2. Slice the beetroots and the avocado on a mandolin to get evenly thick slices. Sprinkle some lemon juice on the avocado to avoid browning.

3. Arrange the beetroot slices in circles on plates.
4. Make the crab salad tarts by pressing the crab meat gently in a small mould (you can use a cookie cutter for this).
5. Place the crab salad in the centre of the beetroot Carpaccio, and arrange some avocado slices around the tarts.

Nutritional values are manually calculated and based on the ingredients specified.
Nutritional value per serving: Calories: 352.7. Fat: 25.4g Saturated Fat: 1.9g Sodium: 16.9 mg. Sugar: 0.0 g
Carbohydrate 35.1g Protein: 3.5 g Dietary fibre: 3.9g

CHARRED ONION, ROASTED PUMPKIN AND BACON SALAD WITH COCONUT CREAM DRESSING

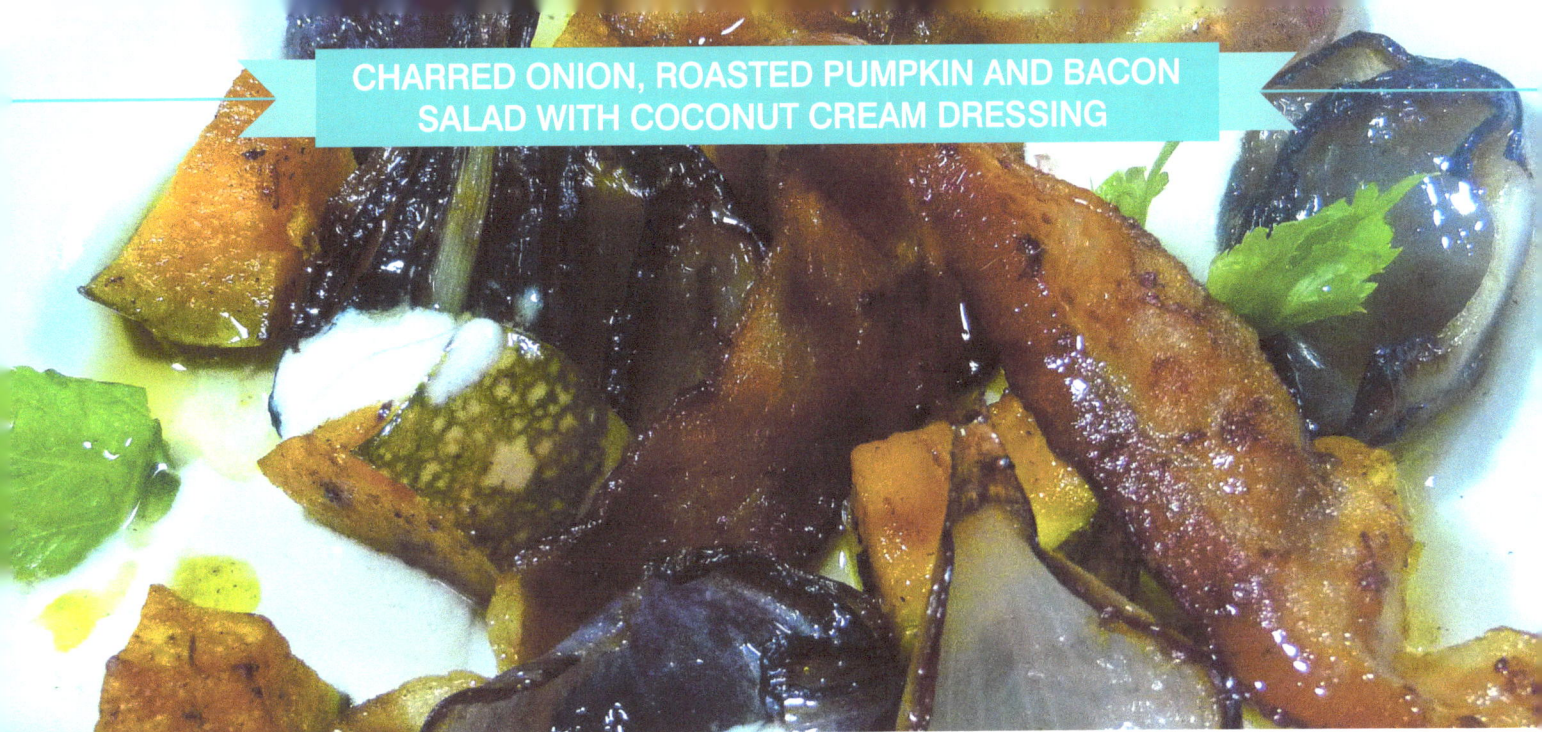

Preparation time: 10 mins

Cooking time: 25 mins

Total time: 35 mins

For me there is nothing like the sweetness and intensified flavours you get from roasting vegetables. A few simple ingredients are all you need to make this delicious salad which proves, once again, that a little extra attention goes a long way.

Ingredients:

Serves 4

- 500gr (1 pound) pumpkin (cut into chunky pieces)
- 8 rashes smoked bacon
- 120gr (4 tbsp) coconut cream
- Pink salt
- 4 small red onions (cut in half)
- 90ml (3 tbsp) olive oil
- Coriander leaves

Method:

1. If you have fresh coconut cream, leave it in the fridge for a day, the cream will coagulate and you can scoop it out. Another way of achieving this is to strain the coconut cream after two days through a cheese cloth, save the milk and use the thick cream for the dressing.
2. Grease a frying pan with a little oil and heat to low/medium heat.
3. Place the onions, cut side down in the pan and fry without moving them for 4 to 5 minutes.
4. Add the pumpkin chunks to the pan plus the remaining oil. You can now move the onions. Give the pan a good shake so all is well mixed.
5. Place the pan in a 180 degree (350 F) pre-heated oven for 20 to 25 minutes.
6. Add the bacon rashes after ten minutes to the pan.
7. When the pumpkin has softened and the bacon is crisp, remove the pan from the oven and allow cooling for 5 minutes.
8. Season the coconut cream and whisk it firmly as you would when whipping cream. When the cream is cold whisking goes really fast, less than a minute.
9. Arrange the salad components on plates. Add some dressing, drizzle a little of the baking oil over the salad, and garnish with coriander leaves.
10. Serve lukewarm.

Nutritional values are manually calculated and based on the ingredients specified.
Nutritional value per serving: Calories: 129.7 Fat: 10.9g Saturated Fat: 2.1g Sodium: 5.4 mg. Sugar: 1.6g Carbohydrate 8.1g Protein: 1.2g Dietary fibre: 1.0g

CLASSIC HUSSAR SALAD WITH GRILLED SARDINES

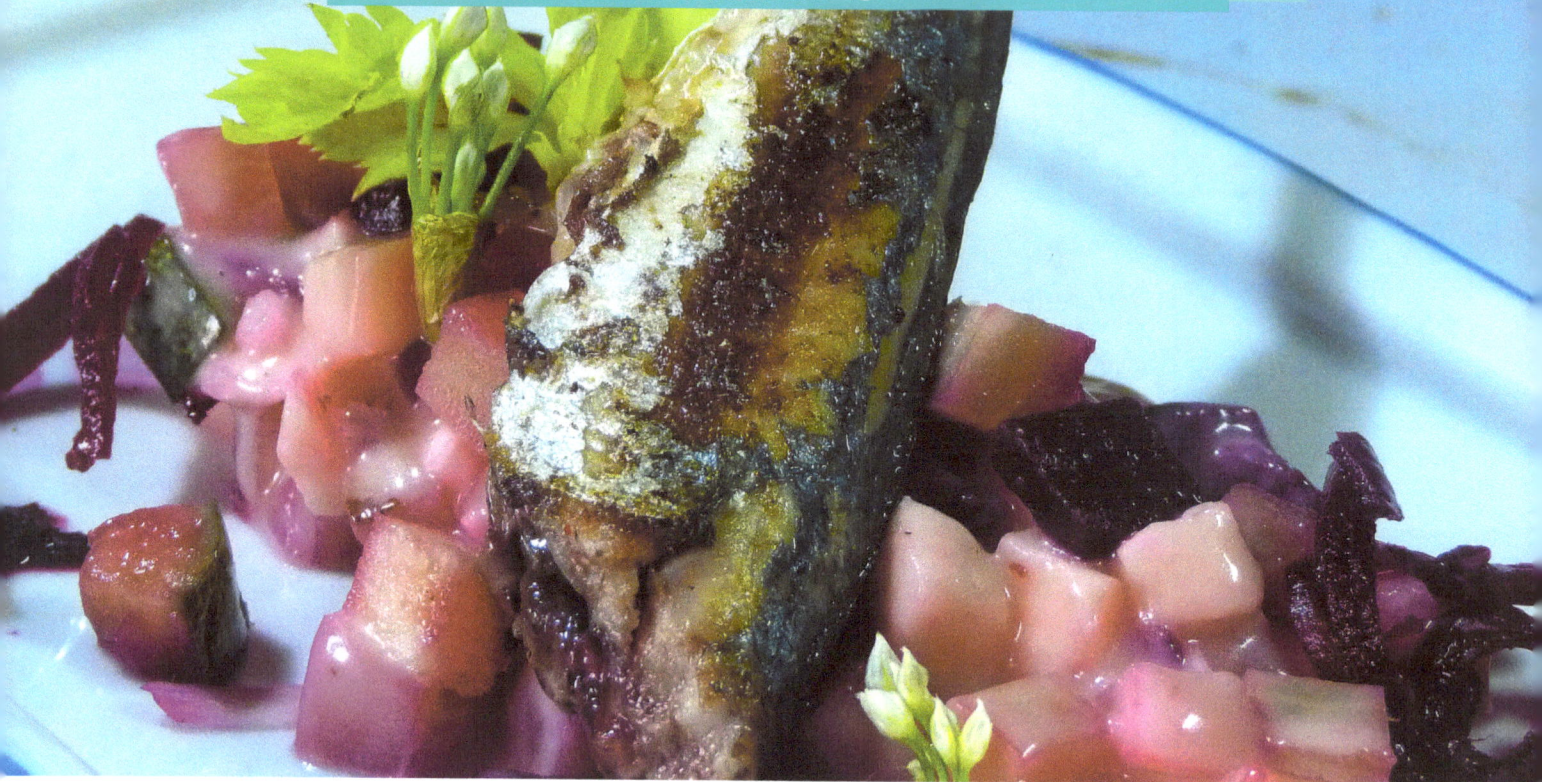

Preparation time: 10 mins

Cooking time: 25 mins

Total time: 35 mins

This classic salad was originally created for soldiers to bring along to the battlefield, a complete meal that could be eaten cold. I gave the salad a little twist to make it AIP warrior friendly, but not less complete.

Ingredients:

Serves 4

- 500gr (1 pound) sweet potato (cut in small dices)
- 120gr (4 tbsp) gherkins (cut in small dices)
- 1 large apple (peeled, cored and cut in small dices)
- 30g (2 tbsp) chopped coriander leaves
- 1 medium onion (finely chopped)
- 90gr (3 tbsp) beetroot pickles (cut in small dices)
- 8 medium sized sardines
- Pink salt

Method:

1. Boil the sweet potato dices in water with a little salt until softened, but still in shape, about 10 minutes.
2. Heat the olive oil in a skillet to medium heat and fry the sardines for 3 to 4 minutes, keep aside.
3. Combine all the ingredients in a bowl, add the mayonnaise and check for taste.
4. Arrange the salad on plates and top with the sardines.
5. Serve cold.

Nutritional values are manually calculated and based on the ingredients specified.
Nutritional value per serving: Calories: 463.4 Fat: 23.0g Saturated Fat: 3.3g Sodium: 576.4mg. Sugar: 3.6g Carbohydrate 54.0g Protein: 8.8g Dietary fibre: 6.2g

GOURMET 'CONFIT' SQUASH SALAD WITH COCONUT RICOTTA

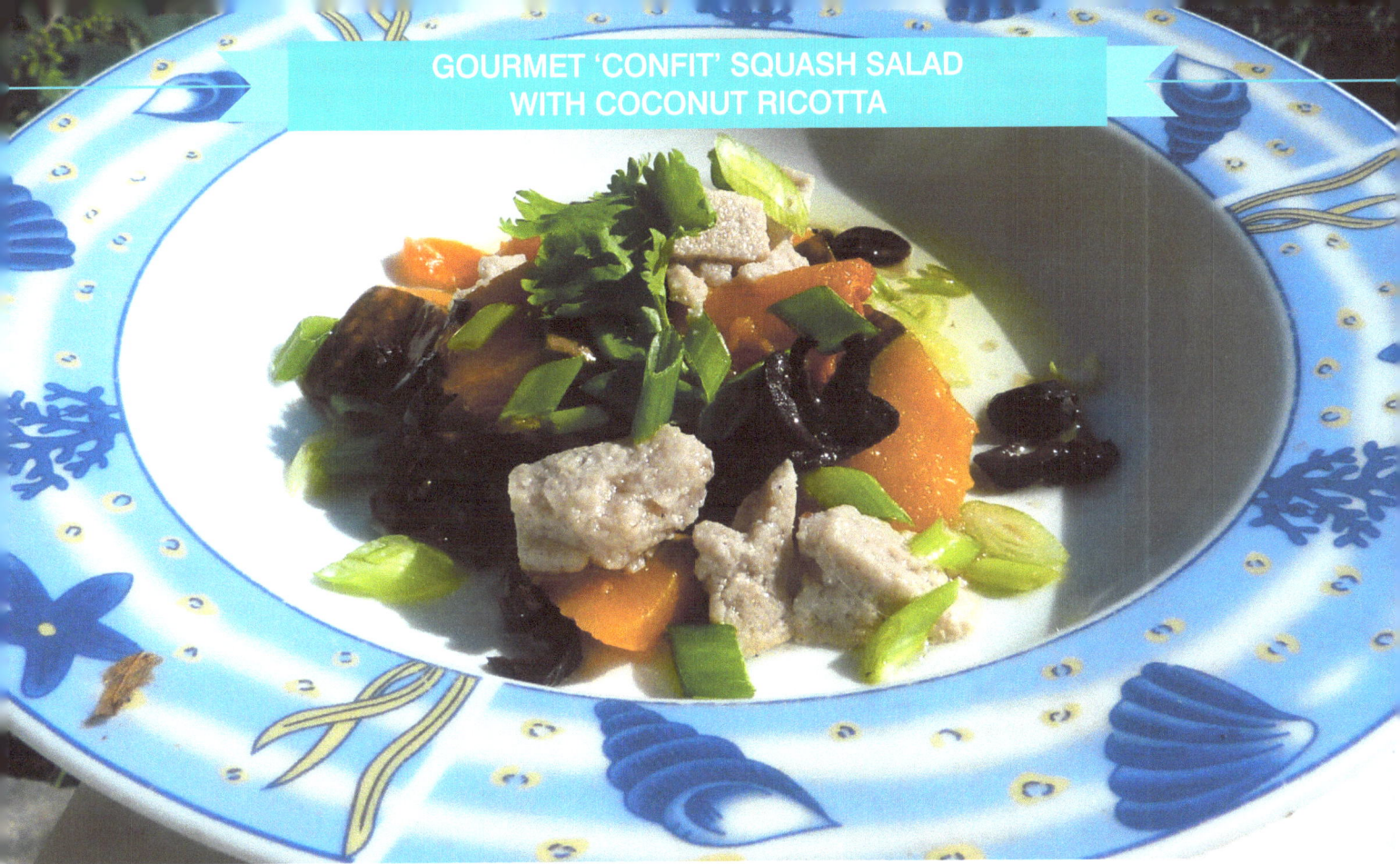

Preparation time: 35 mins	Cooking time: 1 hr 30 mins	Total time: 2 hrs 05 mins

If you are a bit adventurous this may be your thing. Confit is understood by many to be slow cooked duck meat, but 'vegetable confits' are also delicious! Vegetable confits work very well with firm vegetables like carrots and the squash I have used in this recipe. If you can find kabocha squash, great! The skin softens nicely when cooked and you do not need to peel them. Butternut squash works well also, but you need to peel them first. Coconut ricotta is easy and quick to make at home, and has many uses.

Ingredients:

Serves 4

FOR THE CONFIT:

* 1 tsp sea salt * 1 tbsp coconut sugar

* 4 stalks chives * Olive oil

* 500gr (1 pound) Kabocha squash

* 120gr (4 oz) coconut ricotta (homemade, recipe below)

FOR THE RICOTTA:

* 1 Litre (4 cups) coconut cream

* Sea salt

FOR THE DRESSING:

* 125mls (1/2 cup) oil from the confit

* 1 1/2 tbsp lime juice

* 10 black olives (sliced)

Method:

1) To make the ricotta: Bring the coconut cream to a boil on low to medium heat. Boil for 1 to 2 minutes; allow cooling for 10 to 15 minutes.

2) Strain the mix through a cheese cloth, collect the 'whey' and give to your plants.

(3) Hang the cheese cloth so the excess 'whey' can drip out. I hang mine over the sink tap and leave to drip overnight.

(4) Remove from the cloth and season the ricotta with a little salt.

(5) The ricotta is now soft; it will harden quickly when refrigerated, but softens when at room temperature.

(6) To make the confit: Cut the squash in half, then in wedges.

(7) Combine the salt and sugar and coat the squash wedges with this mixture. Leave to marinate, preferably for 30 minutes.

(8) Rinse the squash and cut into bite size pieces.

(9) You need a jar to cook the squash. The size of the jar determines how much oil you need, as you must submerge the squash.

(10) Place the squash in the jar you will use and top with olive oil.

(11) Place the jar in a pot with water so the water reaches the same level as the oil in the jar.

(12) Cook the squash at 85 degrees (185 F) for 1 to 1 ½ hour.

(13) Check if the squash is soft, if not cook a little longer. The timing may vary based on the size of the squash pieces.

(14) Allow to cool and drain the oil. (you can use the oil again)

(15) Combine the dressing ingredients and season as desired.

(16) Divide the squash over 4 individual plates and top with crumbled coconut ricotta, and chopped chives. Lastly drizzle a bit of the dressing around the salad.

(17) Serve slightly warm.

Nutritional values are manually calculated and based on the ingredients specified.
Nutritional value is calculated without the coconut ricotta
Nutritional value per serving: Calories: 212.2 Fat: 12.8g. Saturated Fat: 2.2g. Sodium: 524.5mg. Carbohydrate 19.6g Protein: 3.9g. Dietary fibre: 2.1g.

GREEN MANGO SALAD WITH WATER CRESS AND MANGO DRESSING

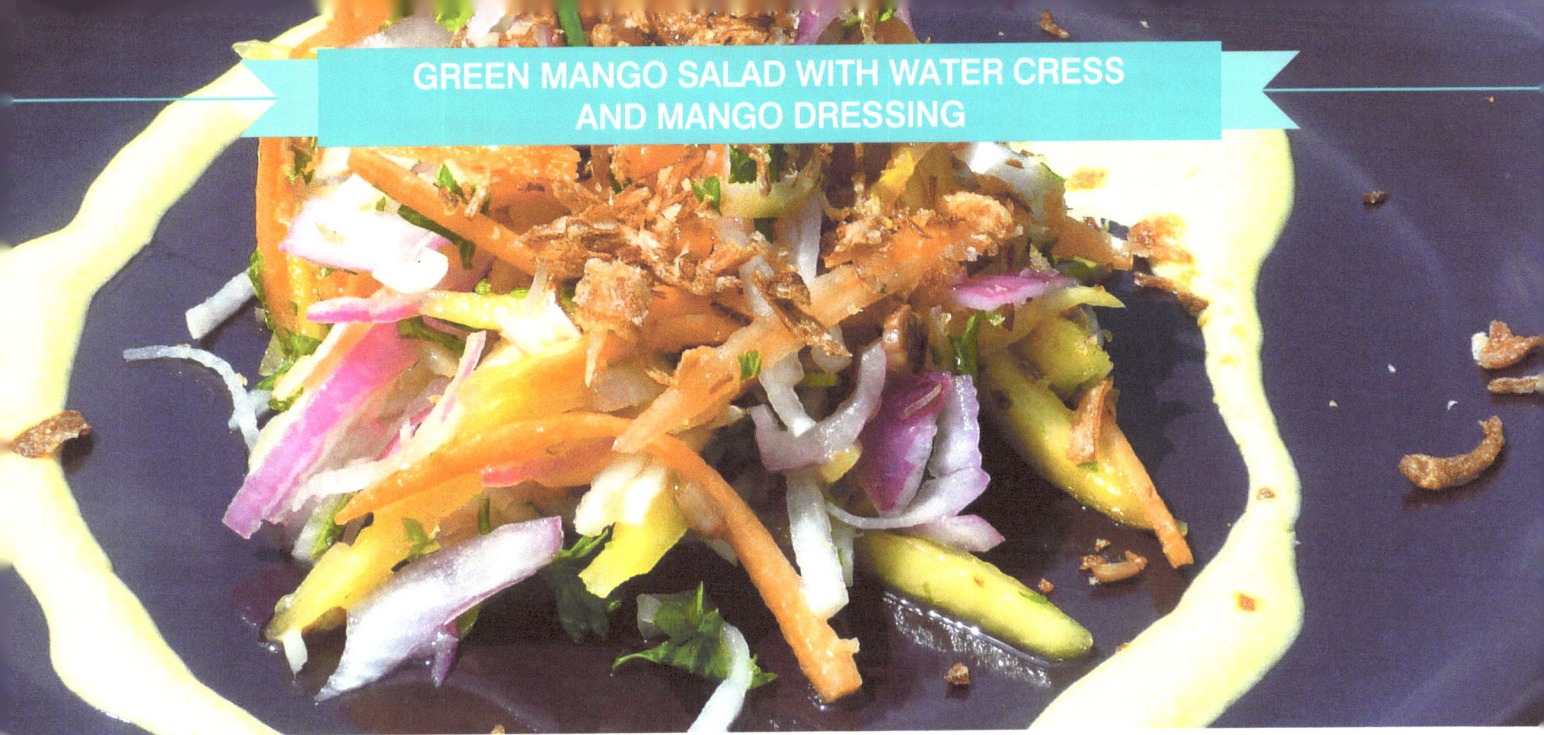

Preparation time: 15 mins	Cooking time: 05 mins	Total time: 20 mins

I love the fresh Asian flavours of this mango salad. A tangy, refreshing salad is always a great addition to seafood dishes. Green mango provides the tang in this salad and the ripe mango gives sweetness. Serve this salad with any seafood dish, but also it works brilliantly with grilled meat as well.

Ingredients: Serves 4

- 15g (1tsp) mint leaves (roughlychopped)
- 1 large green mango
- ½ large carrot (shredded)
- 60ml (2 tbsp) lime juice
- 1 medium onion (sliced in thin half-moon rings)
- 30g (2 tbsp) basil leaves (roughly chopped)

- Pink salt
- 1 bunch of water cress
- 1 large ripe mango
- 125ml (½ cup) olive oil
- ½ large white radish (shredded)
- 2 cloves garlic (minced)
- 30g (2 tbsp) cilantro leaves (roughly chopped)

Method:

1. Before you begin, peel the green mango and cut thin slices from around the seed, place the slices flat and cut them into thin strips.
2. Place the mango strips in a bowl with the carrot, radish, onions and garlic. Add the herbs and mix well.
3. Combine the lemon juice and olive oil in a large bowl and season with salt.
4. Remove the flesh from the ripe mango and blend smooth, the blender will not pick up all the solids. Therefore you need to press the flesh through a fine sieve after blending to get a smooth texture.
5. Divide the water cress into 4 small bundles and cut the stems to size. A good way to hold the bundles together is to tie them with a small rubber band.
6. Toss the salad with enough of the dressing to flavour, do not soak it and allow resting for 10 minutes.
7. Do the same with the water cress bundles.
8. Combine the balance of the dressing with the ripe mango puree.
9. Pipe some mango dressing on individual plates, top with the salad and place a watercress bundle on top (rubber bands removed).

Nutritional values are manually calculated and based on the ingredients specified.
Nutritional value per serving: Calories: 277.1. Fat: 19.5g. Saturated Fat: 2.8g. Sodium: 22.2mg. Carbohydrate 21.5g Protein: 5.6g. Dietary fibre: 9.4g.

GRILLED AVOCADO SALAD WITH SALSA

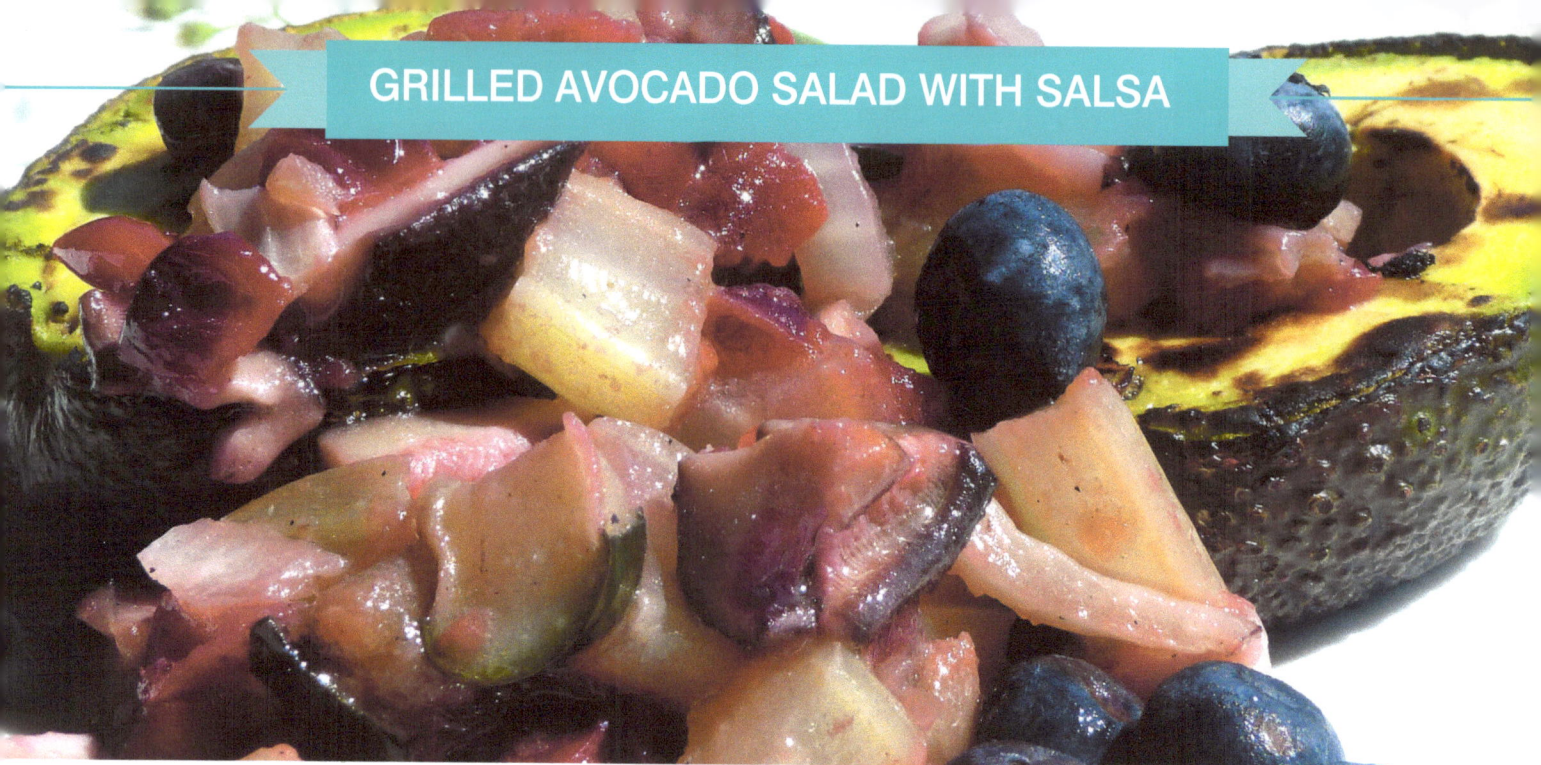

Preparation time: 10 mins

Cooking time: 20 mins

Total time: 30 mins

Avocado is known to be one of the best 'super foods' available. You can eat them whole, in salads, as a dip, in smoothies, the list goes on. Don't be put off by grilled avocados, give it a go! Served with refreshing salsa this is a beautiful looking dish that is so good for you. Be adventurous with the salsa! This is a light refreshing version for all to savour.

Ingredients:

Serves 4

- 125g (4 oz) blueberries
- 125ml (4 oz) pineapple juice
- 30g (2 tbsp) chopped parsley
- 10g (2 tbsp) chopped cilantro
- 1 medium onion (finely sliced)

- Pink salt
- 4 large avocados (skin on, seeds removed)
- 2 cloves garlic (grated)
- 125g (4 oz) mushrooms (chopped)
- 125g (4 oz) celery (sliced)

- 125g (4 oz) cucumber (sliced small)
- 90g (3 tbsp) cranberries
- 10g (1 tbsp) chopped sage
- 60ml (2 tbsp) olive oil
- 125g (4 oz) fennel (finely sliced)

Method:

1. Cut the avocados lengthwise in half, remove the seeds, but leave the skin on.
2. Heat the oil in a skillet to medium heat; add the onion and garlic and fry for 30 seconds.
3. Add the celery, fennel, cucumber and mushrooms and continue frying for another 2 minutes.
4. Add the cranberries and the pineapple juice. Add the herbs, lower the heat and simmer for 10 minutes until all the veggies have softened and combined. Season with a little salt.
5. Pre-heat a grill to 200 degrees (375 F) and grease with a little oil.
6. Place the avocados, flesh side down, on the grill and grill them for 5 minutes.
7. Place the avocado halves on plates, top with the salsa and garnish with the blueberries.

Nutritional values are manually calculated and based on the ingredients specified.
Nutritional value per serving: Calories: 376.5. Fat: 27.1 g. Saturated Fat: 3.7g. Sodium: 44.5mg. Sugar: 13.8g Carbohydrate 35.5g. Protein: 5.4g. Dietary fibre: 14.6g.

SEAFOOD

CRISPY FRIED SARDINES WITH MARINATED FENNEL AND LIME

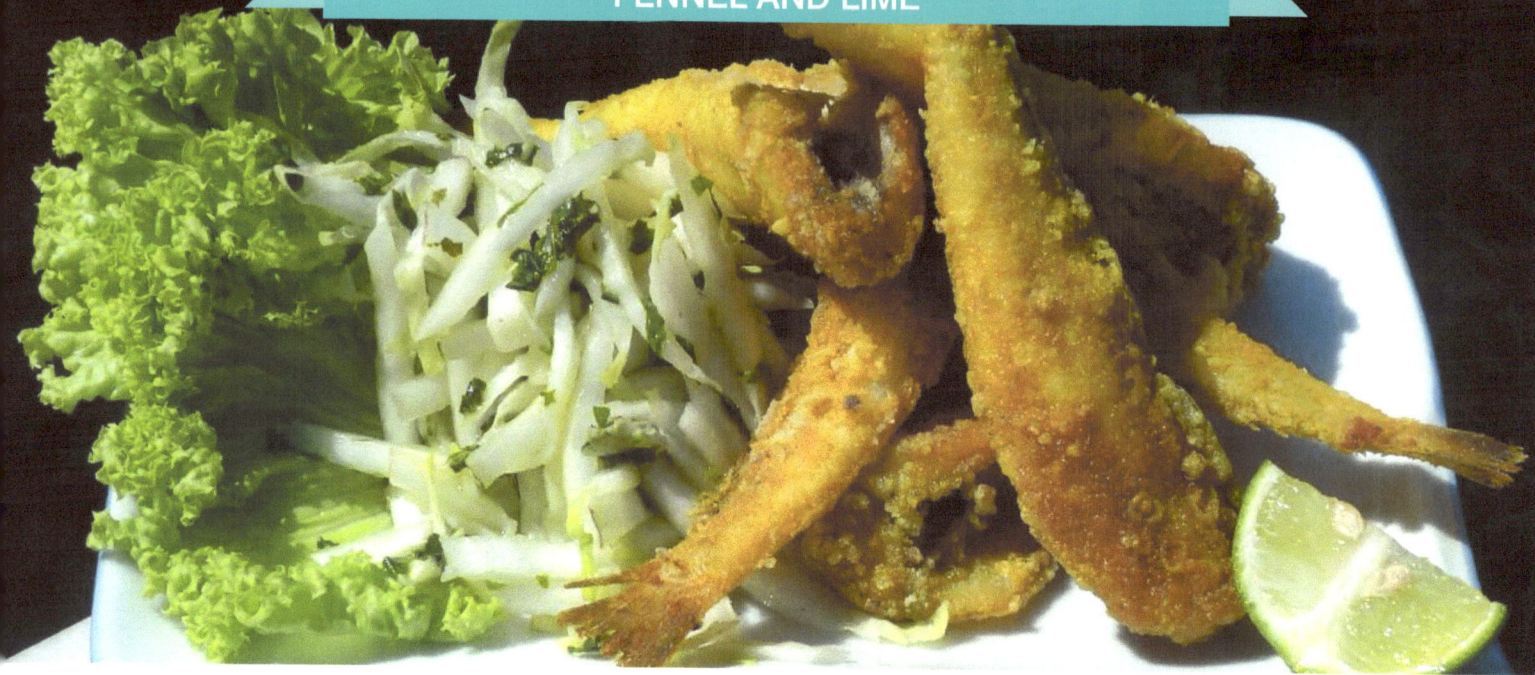

Preparation time: 15 minutes

Cooking time: 5 minutes

Marinating Time: 1 hr

Total time: 1hr 20 minutes

This is a classic combination, there is nothing like seafood with the crisp aromatic flavour of fresh fennel! Use any type of small fish you like. Sardines, sand whiting, or anchovies but make sure to use fresh, sustainable, wild caught fish for this dish. Oily fish has fantastic anti-inflammatory and brain protecting essential Omega 3 fats.

Ingredients: Serves 4

- 16pcs sardines heads removed and gutted (ask your fish monger to do this for you if you like)
- 125g (½ cup) tapioca flour
- 15g (1 tsp) turmeric powder
- 1 fennel bulb

- 10g (1 tsp) tarragon
- 10g (1 tsp) dill   •   90 ml (1 tbsp) olive oil
- Pink salt   •   10g (1 tsp) chervil
- Oil or fat of choice   •   Juice of 1 lime

Method:

1. Cut the fennel bulb in half, remove the core and slice thinly and place in a mixing bowl.
2. Chop the herbs; add to the bowl followed by the lime and oil.
3. Mix well, cover the bowl and allow marinating in the fridge for 1 hour.
4. Combine the tapioca flour with the turmeric and some salt in flat tray or on a plate.
5. Heat the frying oil (palm oil is good for this) in a deep skillet, about 2 cm (1 inch) deep to 180 degrees (325 F).
6. Dip the fish in the flour mix and coat well, hold the fish by the tail and slowly add them to the oil pushing the fish away from you, so you don't get splashed with hot oil.
7. Fry the fish (2 or 3 at a time) for 2 to 3 minutes until golden and crisp, drain on kitchen paper after frying.
8. Arrange the fish on plates with a good scoop of fennel salad and a few lime wedges.

Nutritional values are manually calculated and based on the ingredients specified.
Nutritional value per serving: Calories: 477.9 Fat: 32.8g Saturated Fat: 4.5g Sodium: 324.9 mg. Sugar: 2.0g Carbohydrate 39.7g Protein: 14.9g Dietary fibre: 4.7g

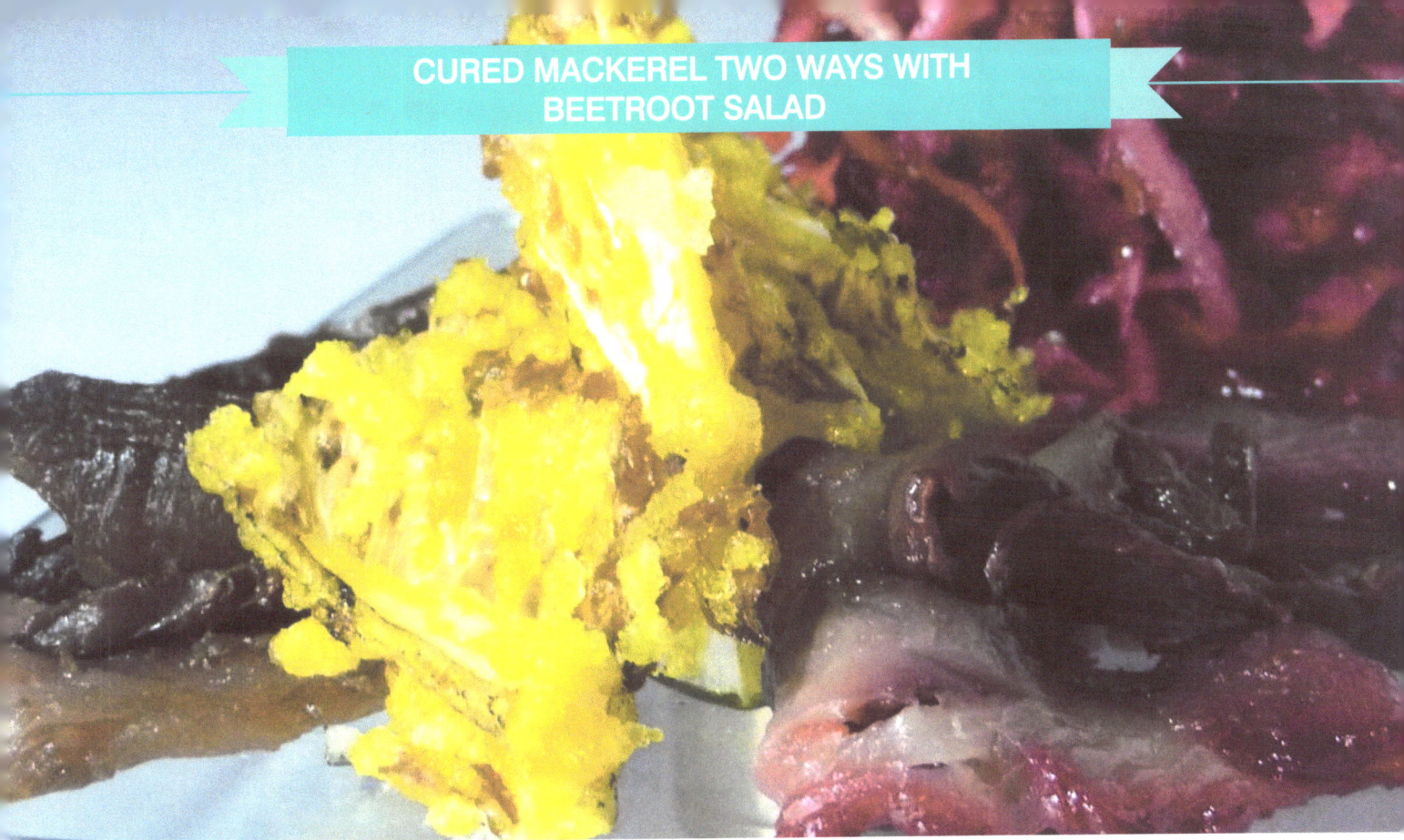

Preparation time: 20 minutes	Cooking time: 10 minutes	Marinating Time: 12 hr	Total time: 12hr 20 minutes

If you thought AIP is boring, try this, invite your friends and give them a 5 Star treat. You can use other fish if you like: salmon, tuna, trevally, I used a small tuna variety

Ingredients: Serves 4

- 120 gr (4 tbsp) raw coconut sugar
- 120 gr (4 tbsp) salt

FOR THE CRISPS:

- 12 pieces of cabbage
- 90 ml cold water

FOR THE FISH:

- About 500 gr (1 pound) skin-less fish fillet, divided into 4 fillets
- 250 gr beet root
- 90 ml (3 tbsp) coconut aminos
- 60 gr (2 tbsp) salt

- Juice of ½ lemon
- 90 ml (3 tbsp) olive oil, Sea salt

- 120gr (4 tbsp) tapioca flour
- Oil for frying

FOR THE SALAD:

- 250 gr (8 oz) beet root (shredded)
- 250 gr (8 oz) apple (shredded)
- 250 gr (8 oz) carrot (shredded)
- 250 gr (8 oz) Swedes or turnips (shredded)

Method:

1. Boil the beet root for 5 minutes in water until slightly softened, drain (keep some of the water) and place in an upright blender, blend smooth. If the blender doesn't pick up the solids add a little cooking water.

2. Add the salt, aminos and sugar.

3. Place the fish fillets two by two in separate containers. Add the beet root mix to one container and cover the other fillets with the salt sugar mix.

4. Cover the fillets with cling wrap and put a little weight on top, I used a small bottle with water

5. Let the fillets with the beetroot juice marinade overnight

6. Let the fillets with the salt sugar mix marinade for 5 hours, wash the salt off the fillets, cover them again, place the weight back and leave to rest in the fridge overnight.

7. Before serving, wash the beetroot from the fillets, return to the fridge to keep cool

8. Heat the oil for the crisps to 180 degrees (325 F)

9. While the oil is heating, combine the tapioca flour with the water add a little salt

10. Combine the salad ingredients

11. Slice the fillets thinly.

12. Dip the cabbage pieces in the batter and fry them in about 1 minute crisp

13. Arrange the fish slices on plates, place some salad on the side and garnish with the cabbage crisps.

Nutritional values are manually calculated and based on the ingredients specified.
Nutritional value per serving: Calories: 397.5. Fat: 7.9 g Saturated Fat: 1.4 g Sodium: 347.0 mg. Sugar: 22.2 g Carbohydrate 52.3 g Protein: 30.8 g Dietary fiber: 4.7 g

FISH BURGER IN SWEET POTATO BUNS

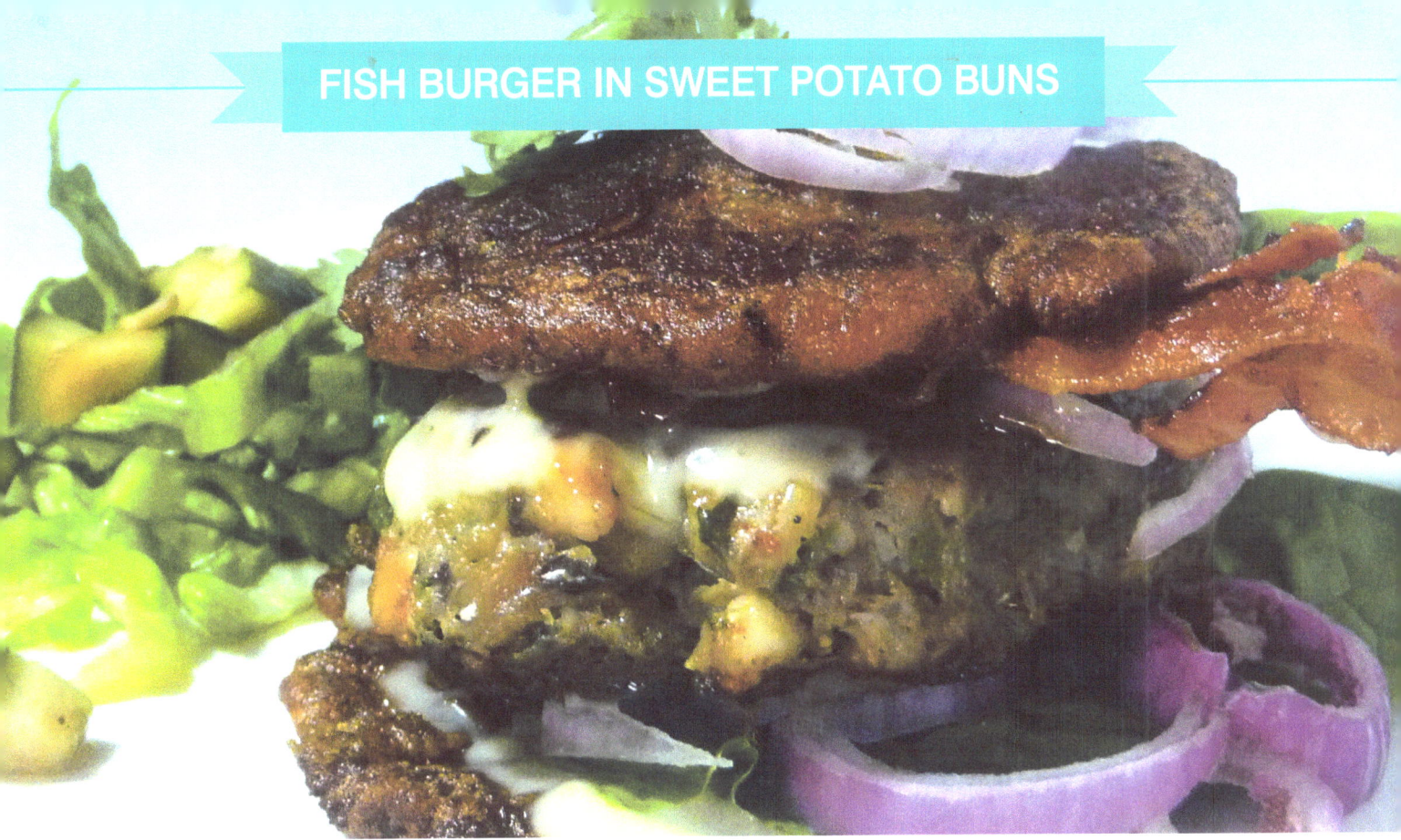

Preparation time: 15 minutes

Cooking time: 25 minutes

Marinating Time: 1 hr

Total time: 1hr 40 minutes

A different twist on the classic chicken burger, simple fast, finger licking good and the kids will love these! The buns not only hold the burgers together but have a great texture too.

Ingredients:

Serves 4

FOR THE BURGER:

- 200gr (6 ½ oz) mackerel
- 200gr (6 ½ oz) pollock
- 200gr (crab meat)
- 200gr (prawn meat)
- 30gr (2 tbsp) chopped dill
- 20gr (1 ½ tsp) bi-carbonate soda

FOR THE SWEET POTATO BUNS:

- 800gr (2 pounds) sweet potatoes (peeled and cut in small pieces)
- 1 medium onion (finely sliced)
- 2 cloves garlic (grated)

- 4 slices bacon
- Pink salt
- 1/2 cup yoghurt mayonnaise
- Half slice red onion
- 1 ½ cups of chopped lettuce of choice
- 1 whole Lebanese cucumber deseeded and roughly chopped

- Oil or fat of choice
- 60gr (2 tbsp) tapioca starch
- Pink salt
- 15gr (1 tbsp) chopped parsley

Method:

1. Chop the fish in small, yet coarse pieces.
   Add the dill, salt and the bi-carb, use your hands to mix all thoroughly, you will notice that the bi-carb functions as a binder that holds the coarse pieces together.

2. Allow the mix to cool in the fridge for 1 hour.

3. Meanwhile cook the sweet potatoes in water with a little salt until fully softened, drain and mash with a potato masher.

4. Add the onion, garlic, parsley, tapioca starch and salt to taste.

5. Allow the mix to cool for about ½ an hour in the fridge.

6. Divide the sweet potato mix into 8 equal portions and roll them into balls.

7. Flatten the balls into round patties of about ¾ cm (1/3 inch) thickness.

8. Heat the oil in a skillet to 180 degrees (350 F) until crispy and golden, about 3 to 4 minutes; drain on kitchen paper and keep aside.

9. Form 4 patties of 200gr each (6 ½ oz) of the fish mix.

10. Grill the patties on a pre-heated grill or on the barbeque, 4 to 5 minutes on each side.

11. Grill the bacon simultaneously.

12. Spread some yoghurt mayonnaise on a sweet potato patty, top with a lettuce leaf and some sliced onion. Place a fish patty on top, followed by some more mayonnaise, lettuce, onion and cucumber.

13. Top the burger with a slice of bacon and a second sweet potato patty.

14. Serve hot.

Nutritional values are manually calculated and based on the ingredients specified.
Nutritional value per serving: Calories: 736.9 Fat: 40.8g Saturated Fat: 7.9g Sodium: 1082.8mg. Sugar: 0.0g Carbohydrate 38.9g Protein: 52.0g Dietary fibre: 3.9g

MARINATED BLACK COD WITH BRAISED WOMBOK

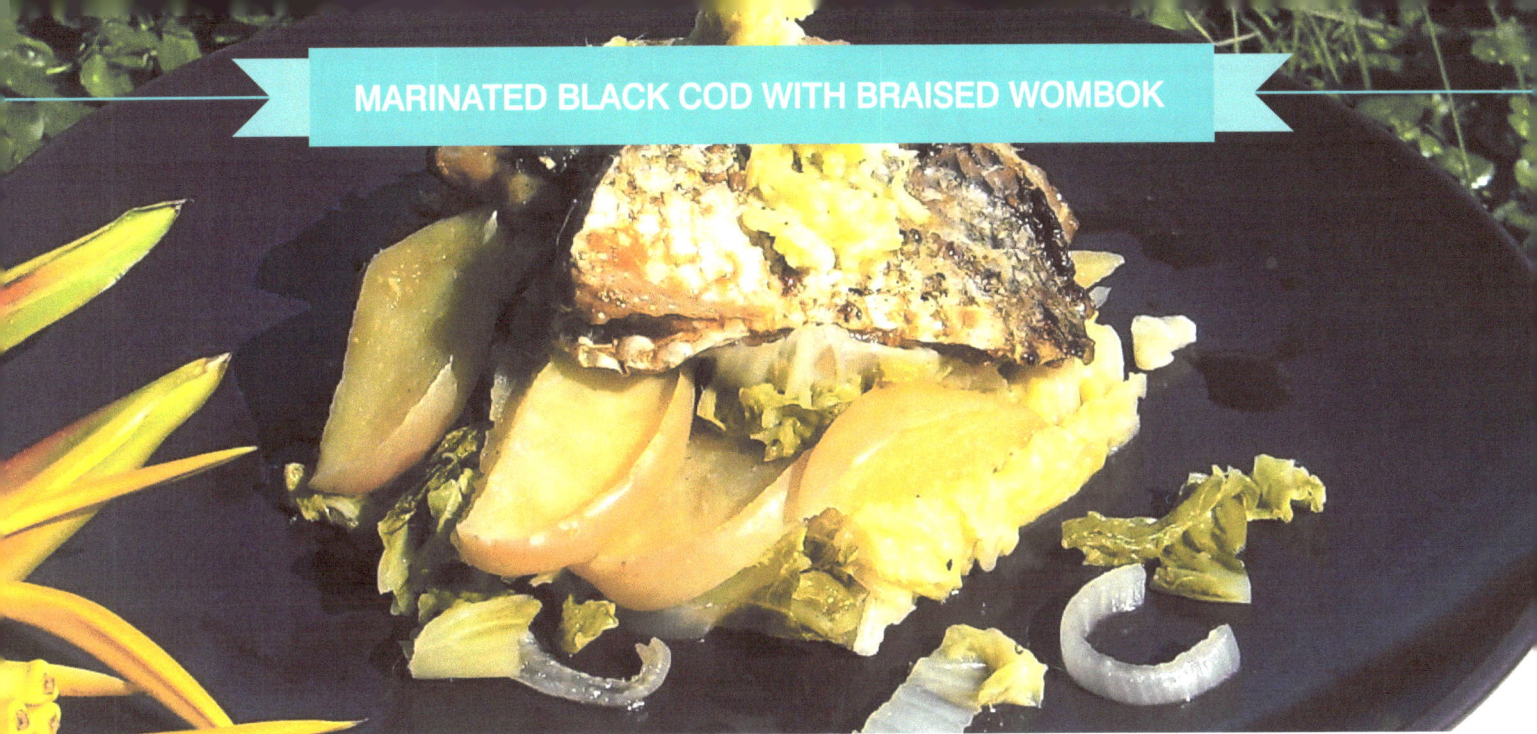

Preparation time: 20 minutes

Cooking time: 40 minutes

Marinating Time: 2 hrs

Total time: 3 hrs

One of my favourite things in the world to eat is crispy skinned fish. Whilst working in restaurants I would often clear plates with the beautiful crispy fish skin discarded to the side of the plate! It may not be the ideal food sensation for everyone, but to me it's the best bit and highly nutritious. Black cod is rich in protein and polyunsaturated Omega 3 fatty acids, both so important to healing, and the subtle sweetness of the wombok and apple work really well with this dish.

Ingredients: Serves 4

• FOR THE BLACK COD

• Juice of ½ a lemon

• 60gr (2 tbsp) grated ginger

• 4 Black cod fillets (skin-on, 180gr (6 oz) each or similar deep sea oily fish with skin on

• 30ml (1 tbsp coconut amino)

• 1 stalk lemon grass (finely sliced)

• 60ml (2 tbsp olive oil)

• FOR THE WOMBOK:

• 600g (1 ½ pound) wombok (cut in 5 cm (2 inch) pieces

• 1 medium onion (sliced)

• 2 cloves garlic

• 1 apple (peeled cored and cut in slices)

• 125ml (½ cup) bone broth

Method:

1. Place the cod fillets in a bowl, add the marinade ingredients mix and cover the bowl, allow marinating for two hours or overnight.

2. Pre- heat an oven to 125 degrees (257 F).
3. Place the wombok in a rimmed saucepan; spread the onion, garlic and apple over the cabbage, top with bone broth and a pinch of salt. Simmer for 25 to 30 minutes on low heat.
4. Heat the olive oil in a skillet until very hot; remove the cod fillets from the marinade and pat dry with kitchen paper.
5. Fry the cod skin down for 3 minutes on high, flip them over and lower the heat to medium, fry for another 2 minutes.
6. Divide the wombok over plates, top with cod fillet skin side up, and garnish with the cabbage crisps.

Nutritional values are manually calculated and based on the ingredients specified.
Nutritional value per serving: Calories: 336.6 Fat: 10.8g Saturated Fat: 1.7g Sodium: 411.0mg Carbohydrate 15.2g Protein: 42.9g Dietary fibre: 5.0g

OVEN BAKED MUSSELS WITH BACON

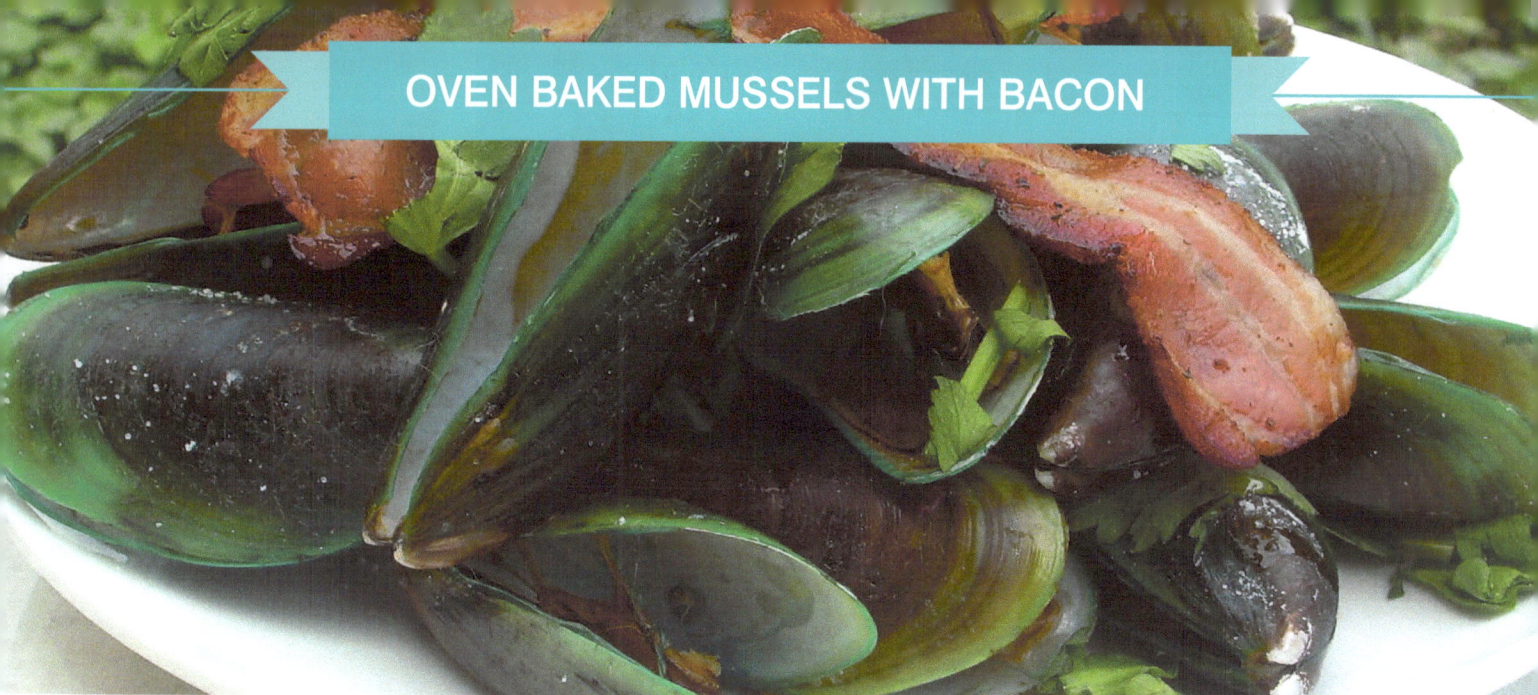

Preparation time:
15 mins

Cooking time:
15 mins

Total time:
30 mins

Hands down one of my favourite seafood's are mussels, the salty ocean taste with all those mouth watering juices and perfectly tender little morsels inside! Magnifique! Only after cooking for some time did I learn that oven baking mussels is something to explore. This classic combo of bacon and mussels is heaven; smokey crunchy bacon makes the whole dish quite special.

Ingredients:

Serves 4

- 2kg (4 lbs) mussels in shell
- 12 rashes smoked streaky bacon
- 125g (1/2 cup) sliced onion
- 30g (2 tsp) salt

- Good handful of chopped celery leaves
- 60g (2 tbsp) chopped garlic
- 30g (1tbsp) olive oil

Method:

1. Pre-heat an oven to 250 Celsius (400 F)
2. Wash and de-beard the mussels under running water for 10 minutes if you don't have mussels that have already been cleaned.

3. Meanwhile heat the olive oil in a large skillet to medium heat and fry the bacon crispy.
4. Drain the bacon on kitchen paper, preserve the fat.
5. Strain the mussels of all water and spread them over a rimmed baking tray.
6. Sprinkle the onion, garlic, preserved fat and salt over the mussels and bake them for 15 minutes in the oven, or until they have all opened.
7. Discard any mussels that have not opened and transfer to a serving dish.
8. Top with the crispy bacon and garnish with celery leaves.

Nutritional values are manually calculated and based on the ingredients specified.
Nutritional value per serving (12 slices per cake): Calories: 388.3 Fat: 15.0g Saturated Fat: 3.5g Sodium: 1549.7mg Carbohydrate 12.6g Protein: 46.6g Dietary fibre: 0.4g

PAN FRIED SEA BASS FILLET WITH SPINACH AND SWEET POTATO PUREE

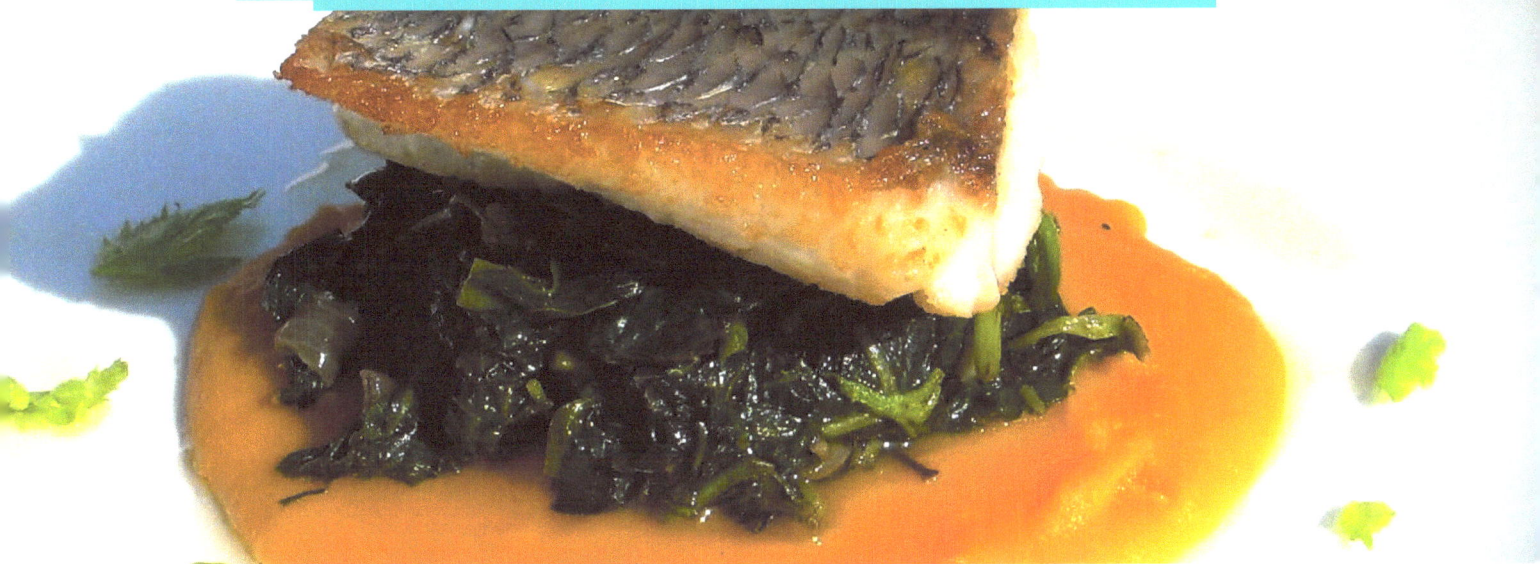

Preparation time: 10 mins

Cooking time: 15 mins

Total time: 25 mins

Sea bass is a lovely white fish to eat; in this quick and easy recipe we combine the fish with iron rich spinach and orange sweet potato. This is another great dish to get fish into your diet.

Ingredients:

Serves 4

- 600g (1 ¼ lbs) skin-on sea bass fillet
- 1 kg (2 lbs) baby spinach
- 600g (2 ¼ cups) orange sweet potatoes
- 75ml (1/4 cup) coconut butter

- 90g (3 tbsp) olive oil • Sea salt
- 60g (2 tbsp) chopped onion
- 3 cloves garlic, 2 finely chopped
- 60g (2 tbsp) lemon juice

Method:

1. Peel and wash the sweet potato and cut into pieces.
2. Boil the sweet potato wedges in water with a little salt, and the whole garlic clove until they are soft, about 10 minutes. Drain and allow cooling for a few minutes.
3. Transfer to an up-right blender, add the coconut butter and blend until smooth. Transfer back to the pan and adjust the thickness if needed.
4. Heat 2/3 of the olive oil in a large skillet to medium heat, add the onions and chopped garlic, fry for 1 minute and add the spinach. Fry until wilted and soft, about 5 minutes. Add a little water during the process to cook the spinach through.
5. Drain the spinach in a sieve or colander to allow excess water to drain out.
6. Chop the spinach roughly, add the coconut butter and mix through.
7. Heat the left over oil in a non-stick frying pan on high heat, season the sea bass fillet with salt and fry skin-side down for about 3 minutes. Flip over and continue frying for another 2 minutes. Timing may vary based on the thickness of the fillet, but ensure not to overcook.
8. Remove the fillets from the pan, add the lemon juice.
9. Place some sweet potato puree on plates, top with spinach and a piece of sea bass and drizzle some of the lemon juice around it.

Nutritional values are manually calculated and based on the ingredients specified.
Nutritional value per serving: Calories: 485.3 Fat: 12.4g. Saturated Fat: 3.0g. Sodium: 106.7mg. Carbohydrate 30.6g. Protein: 73.1g. Dietary fibre: 2.1g.

PAN SEARED WHITE FISH WITH OLIVES, CAPERS, ANCHOVIES AND GRILLED LETTUCE

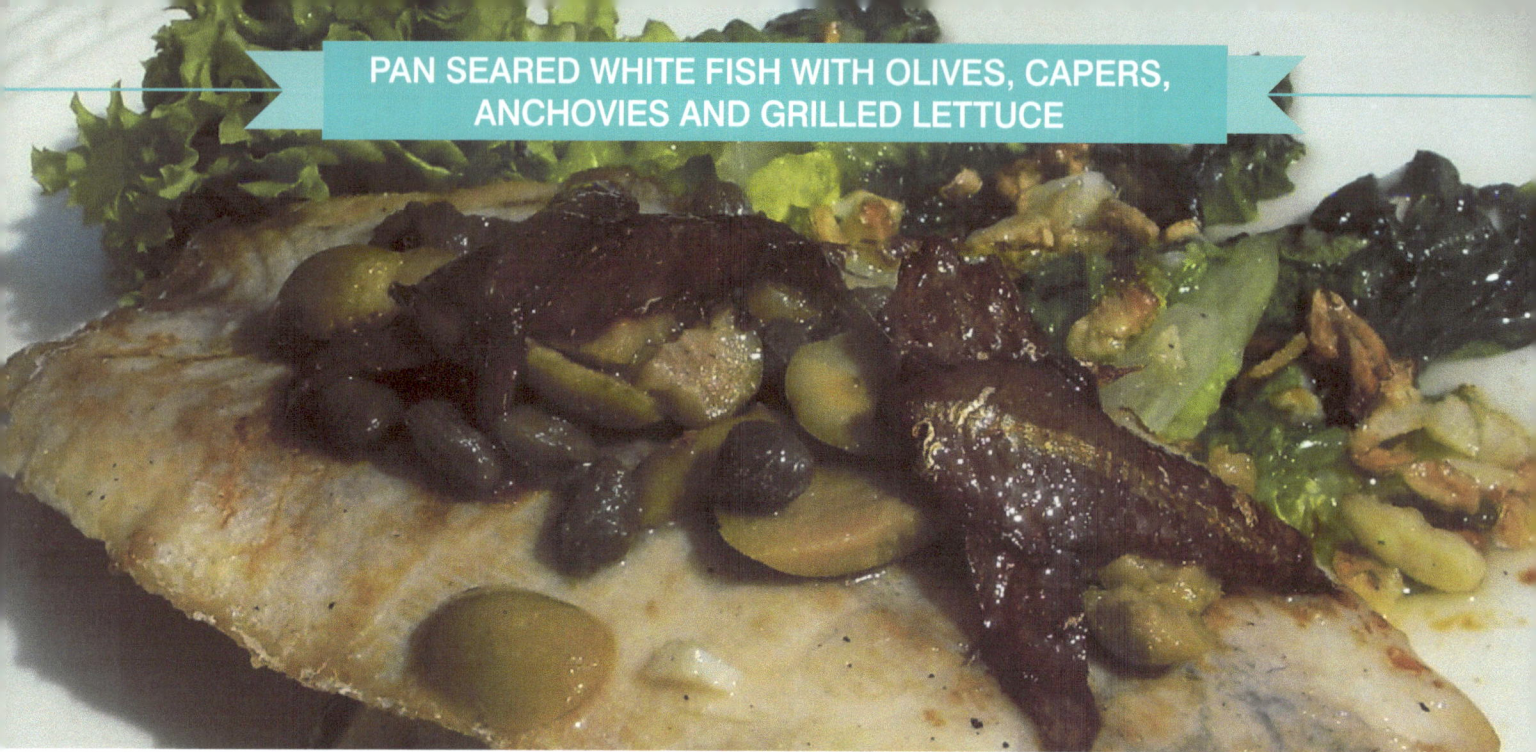

Preparation time: 10 mins

Cooking time: 10 mins

Total time: 20 mins

If simplicity is the key then this dish must be about the ultimate experience. Delicious fish, perfectly grilled vegetables, and a salty tangy garnish. It doesn't get much better than that. Experiment with different types of lettuces, you will be surprised how well grilled lettuce works in this dish.

Ingredients: Serves 4

- 60gr (2 tbsp) lemon juice
- 60gr (2 tbsp) capers
- 8pcs anchovy fillet
- 450gr lettuce (sliced lengthwise in half)

- 60gr (2 tbsp) chopped garlic • Pink sea salt
- 125 ml (1/2 cup) olive oil
- 60gr (2 tbsp) kalamata olives (sliced)tt
- 4 white fish fillets of your choice, (about 200gr (6 ½oz) each

Method:

1. Spread the fish fillets out on a tray and season with salt and half of the lemon juice.
2. Spread the lettuce leaves on another tray, sprinkle with olive oil and rub the garlic up and between the leaves.
3. Heat a grill or griddle to medium heat, and grill the lettuce for 2 to 3 minutes on both sides.

4. Heat a skillet with some olive oil on high heat, and fry the fish fillets 2 minutes on each side. Add the capers and olives followed by the remaining lemon juice. Turn off the heat.

5. Arrange the lettuce leaves on plates and top with the fillets, scoop the olive/ caper juice over it. Lastly, place two anchovy fillets on each plate and serve.

Nutritional values are manually calculated and based on the ingredients specified.
Nutritional value per serving: Calories: 238.6. Fat: 5.1g Saturated Fat: 0.5g Sodium: 1193.1mg Carbohydrate 3.5g Protein: 44.7g Dietary fibre: 2g

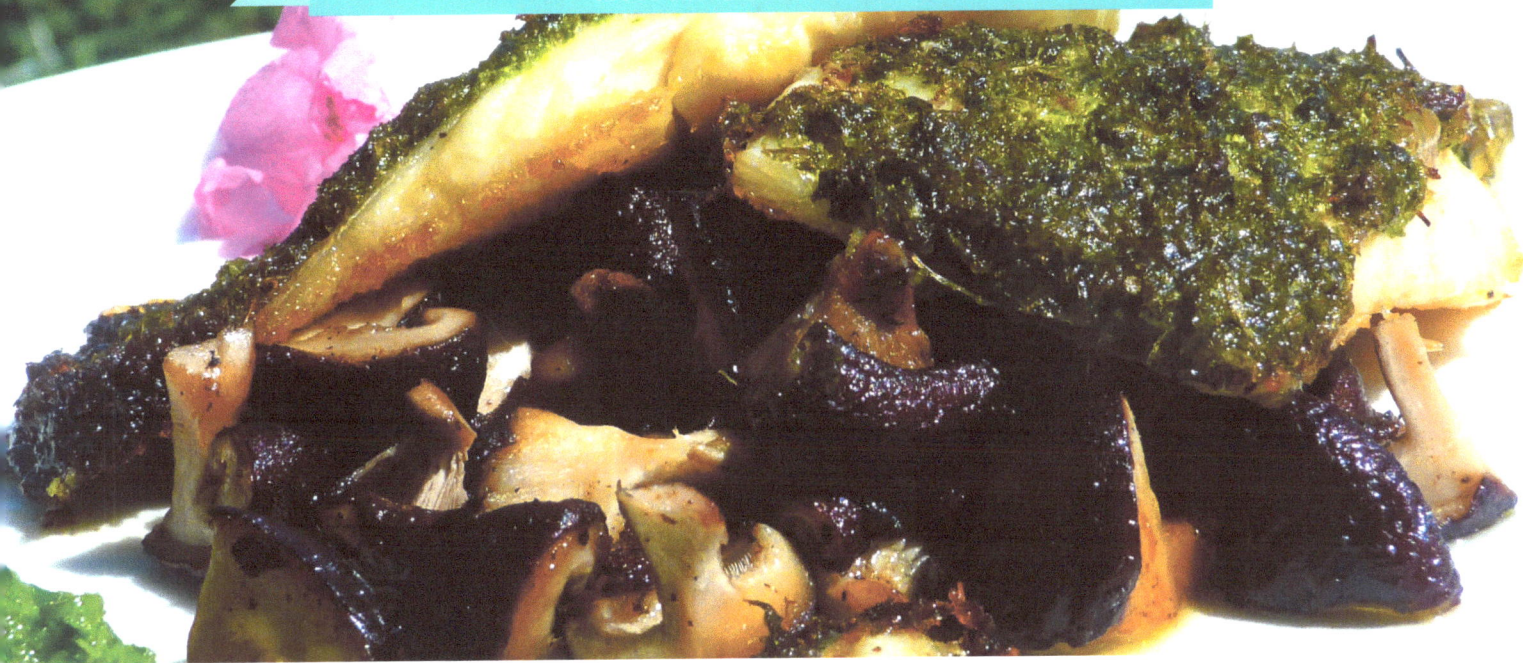

PESTO INFUSED RED SNAPPER WITH MUSHROOMS

Preparation time: 20 mins

Cooking time: 15 mins

Total time: 35 mins

Red Snapper is a typical game fish with meaty flesh, low in fat but high in vitamins D and E. Red snapper is a delicious fish to have on your plate. The fish will come in various sizes, so you have to adjust the portion sizes a bit at times, however that doesn't make them less tasty. The snapper is combined in this recipe with pesto and lovely fried mushrooms, with lemon for some zing making this a definite palate pleaser.

Ingredients:
Serves 4

FOR THE PESTO:
- 4 brown shallots (cut in quarters)
- 2 garlic cloves • 1 tbsp fresh squeeze lemon juice
- 100g (1cup) fresh basil leaves
- ¼ cup olive oil • Pink salt to taste

FOR THE RED SNAPPER:
- 600g (1 ½ pound) skin on red snapper fillet
- 60ml (2 tbsp) lemon juice • 60g (2 tbsp) olive oil
- 400g (14 oz) Shi-Take mushrooms

Method:

1. To make the pesto: heat a skillet to medium heat; add the shallots and garlic and fry to brown them in 2 to 3 minutes.
2. Place the browned shallots and garlic in an up-right blender. Add the basil leaves and turn the blender on slowly, add the olive oil until you get a slightly coarse mixture, season with a little salt. Transfer to a container.
3. Score the skin of the snapper with a sharp knife by making small incisions about 1 cm (1/2 inch) apart.
4. Rub the lemon juice and a little salt in the incisions and spread pesto over it until covered.
5. Pre-heat oven to 180 (325 F) degrees.
6. Heat the olive oil in a skillet to medium hot, add the mushrooms and fry for a minute, transfer the mushrooms to a baking tray and top with the snapper fillets, skin-side up.
7. Bake in the oven for 12 to 15 minutes, depending on the thickness of the fillets. If you can easily pierce a small knife through the fillets they are cooked.
8. Divide over plates and serve with lemon wedges.

Nutritional values are manually calculated and based on the ingredients specified.
Nutritional value per serving: Calories: 416.9 Fat: 23.3g. Saturated Fat: 3.5g. Sodium: 100.2mg. Carbohydrate: 3.6g. Protein: 46.7g. Dietary fibre: 1.4g.

PRAWN AND VEGETABLE TEMPURA

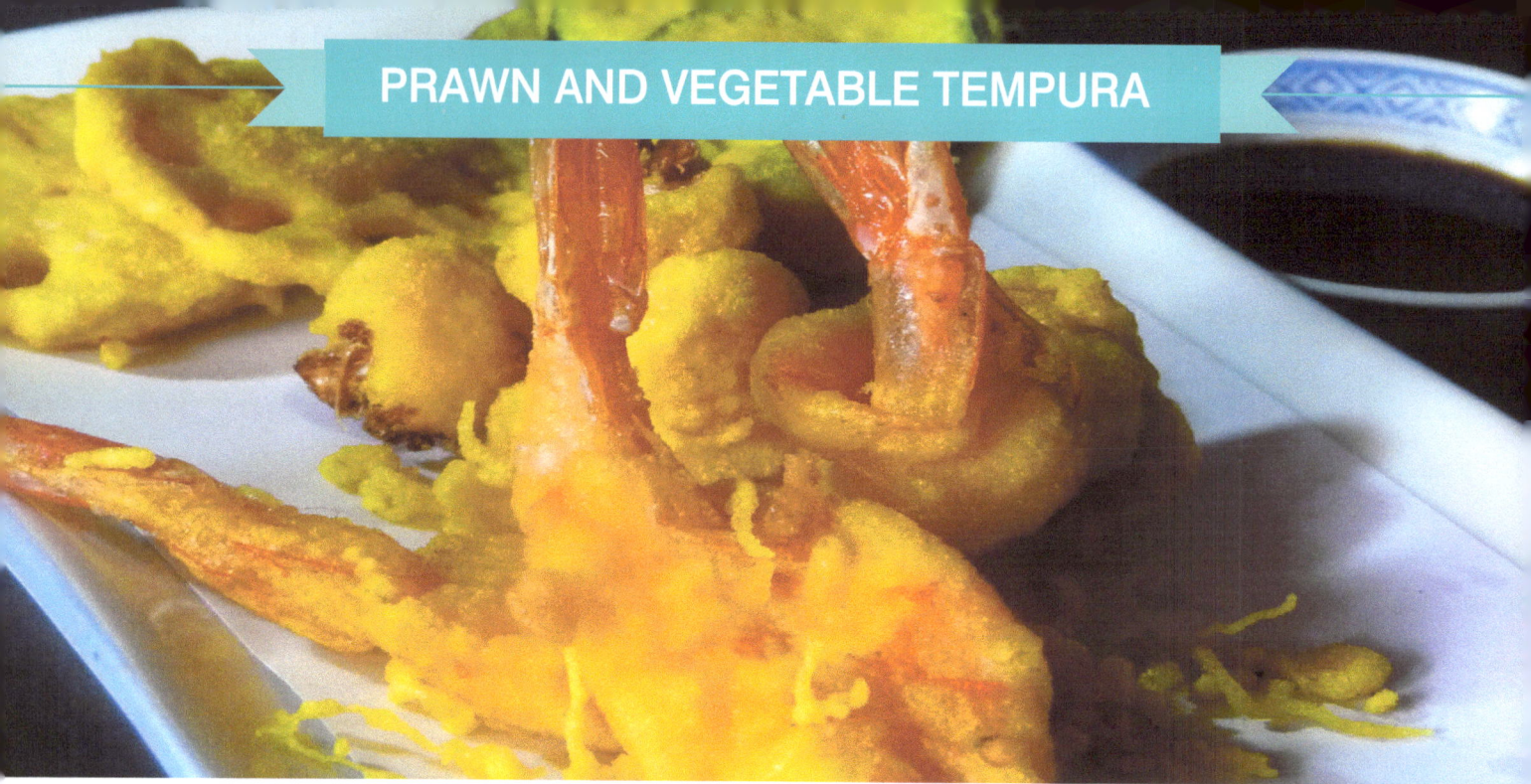

Preparation time: 15 mins

Cooking time: 10 mins

Total time: 25 mins

Growing up, Japanese cuisine was one of my favourite foods. Tempura is a great way to get that crunch back in your AIP diet! Tapioca flour gives a lovely crisp finish when deep fried, so why not take advantage of this feature and indulge in this Japanese favourite? Served with a dip of coconut amino it makes a delicious starter or snack. Tapioca flour does not colour very well when fried, so I added a pinch of turmeric powder for a golden finish.

Ingredients: Serves 4

FOR THE BATTER:
* 250gr (1 cup) tapioca flour
* 90ml (3 oz) cold water
* 5gr (½ tsp) turmeric powder
* Oil for frying • Little Pink salt

FOR THE TEMPURA:
* 12 small broccoli or cauliflower florets
* 12 slices zucchini • 12 small mushrooms
* 12 medium sized prawns

Method:

① Place the tapioca flour in a bowl with a little salt and sprinkle the water evenly over the flour.
② Use your fingers to combine the flour with the water, so you get a batter like texture.
③ Heat the oil to 180 degrees (350 F).
④ Dip the individual pieces of ingredients in to the batter, and then dip them slowly in the oil.
⑤ Dip first half way so the frying starts, release after a few seconds, this will prevent the individual pieces sticking together.
⑥ Fry all ingredients bit by bit for the best result, and drain on a rack or kitchen paper.
⑦ Lastly drizzle some of the remaining batter in the oil for garnish.
⑧ Serve the tempura on a sheet of paper with a coconut amino dip.

Nutritional values are manually calculated and based on the ingredients specified.
Nutritional value per serving: Calories: 162.1 Fat: 0.7g Saturated Fat: 0.1g Sodium: 323.6mg. Sugar: 3.0g Carbohydrate 34.4g Protein: 6.6g Dietary fibre: 3.0g

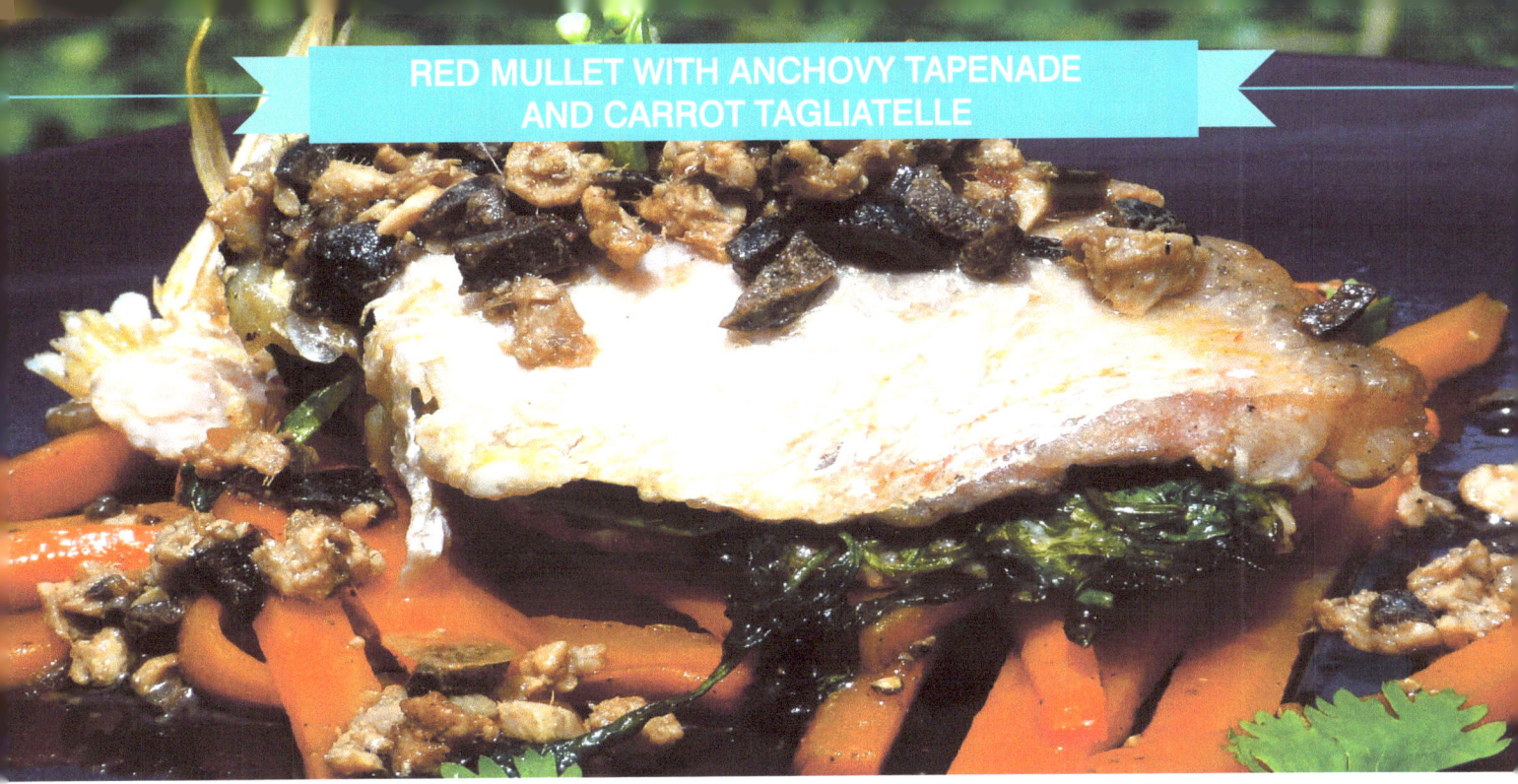

RED MULLET WITH ANCHOVY TAPENADE AND CARROT TAGLIATELLE

Preparation time: 20 mins

Cooking time: 10 mins

Total time: 30 mins

Red mullet is a lovely flaky fish, a Mediterranean favourite that combines well with anchovies and olives. Sweet 'Al Dente' cooked carrot compliments the dish very well.

Ingredients:

Serves 4

FOR THE BATTER:

- 8 red mullet fillets skin-on (250gr, 8 oz) per 2 fillets
- 2 limes (cut in slices)
- 4 sprigs coriander leaves
- 12 black olives   • Juice of 1 lime
- 60ml (2 tbsp) olive oil
- 600g (1 ½ pounds) carrot
- Pink salt
- 8 anchovy fillets

Method:

1. Slice the carrots lengthwise on a mandolin into thin slices, or place them flat on a chopping board and cut lengthwise ½ cm (¼ inch) broad tagliatelle strips.
2. Cook the tagliatelle in water with a bit of salt for 3 to 4 minutes, drain and rinse cold.
3. Chop the anchovies and the olives finely.
4. Arrange the mullet fillets on a tray, divide the lime slices on the meat side over one half of the fillets, top with a sprig of coriander and top with another fillet half, meat side down , press a bit so they stick together.
5. Heat the olive oil in a skillet to high heat, sprinkle a little salt on the skin of the fillets and carefully add them to the pan.
6. Fry for 2 minutes and turn them over with a spatula, fry for another 2 minutes.
7. Remove from the pan and keep aside.
8. Add the anchovies/olives mix (tapenade) to the pan, fry for 30 seconds, and add the lime juice. Remove from the pan and keep aside.
9. Now add the tagliatelle to the pan and fry for a few minutes, season with salt.
10. Arrange some tagliatelle on plates, top with a mullet sandwich and top with the tapenade.
11. Serve hot.

Nutritional values are manually calculated and based on the ingredients specified.
Nutritional value per serving: Calories: 613.5. Fat: 38.3g Saturated Fat: 4.7g Sodium: 867.9mg. Sugar: 6.9g Carbohydrate 15.4g Protein: 49.8g Dietary fibre: 4.7g

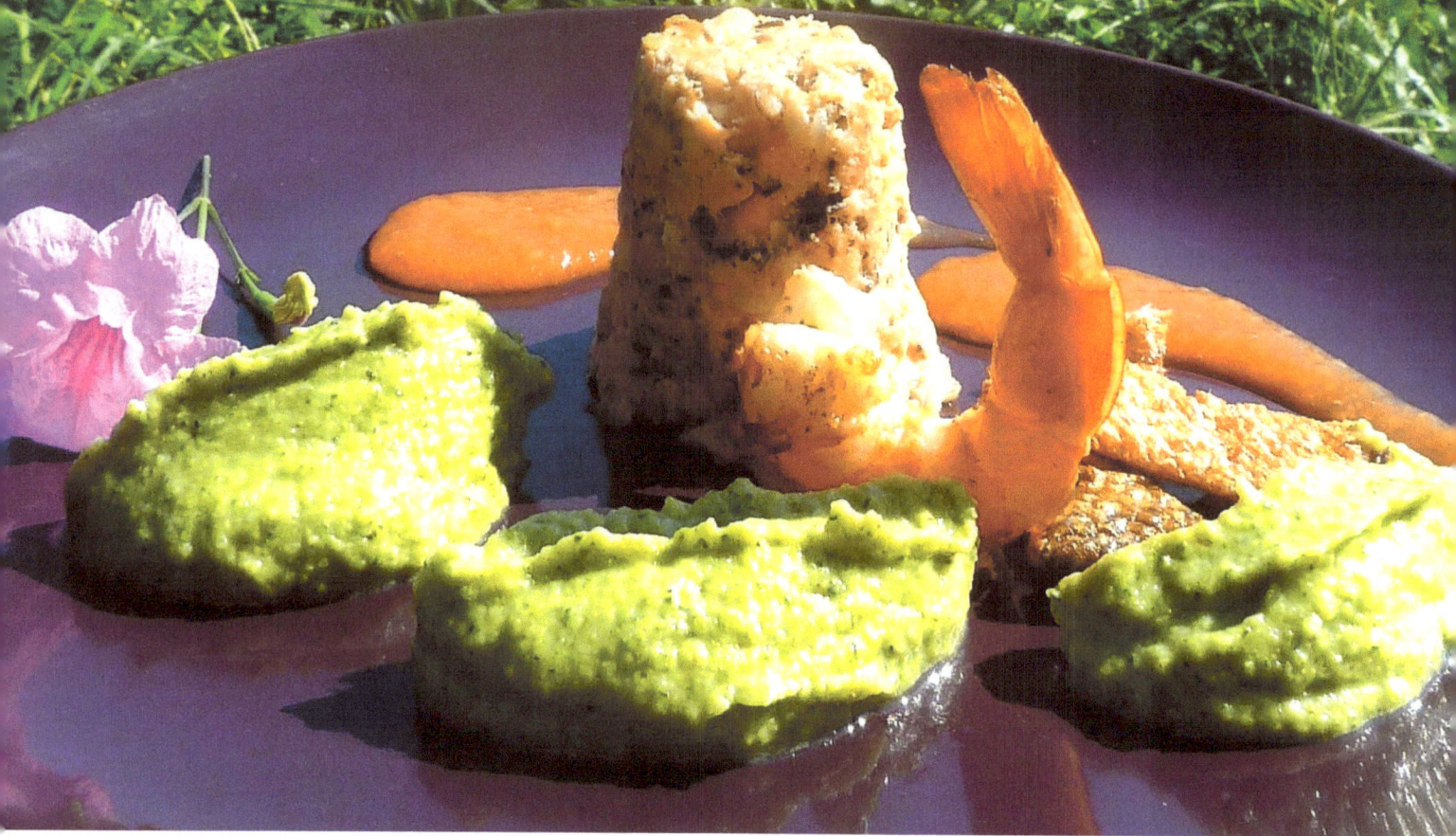

Preparation time: 30 mins

Cooking time: 30 mins

Total time: 60 mins

Salmon is a very versatile fish that can be used for many recipes, high in Omega 3 and fatty acids that are key nutrients in your healing. There are some great textures happening in this dish, the sweet papaya and seafood is another classic combination. Salmon also combines very well with prawns, which this recipe reveals.

Ingredients:

Serves 4

- 450g (1 pound) salmon fillet
- 150g (5 oz) peeled prawns (4 with tail intact)
- 600g (1 ½ pound) broccoli chopped into florets including stem
- 250g (1 cup) papaya
- 30ml (1 tbsp) olive oil

- 60g (2 tbsp lime juice)
- 125ml (1/2 cup coconut milk)
- Zest of 1 lime
- 30g (2 tbsp) fresh dill
- Sea salt

Method:

1. Cut the salmon into small pieces and place in an up-right blender, add the dill, lime zest and a little salt. Turn the blender on and slowly add the coconut milk until you have a smooth, slightly firm consistency. You may not use all of the coconut milk.

2. Remove from the blender and place in a bowl. Chop the peeled prawns by hand until slightly coarse, add the prawns to the salmon and combine.

3. Using the whole of the broccoli, the stem has very tasty flesh, boil in water with a little salt until soft, about 10 minutes. Drain and allow cooling for 2 minutes.

4. While the broccoli is cooking, blend the papaya with the lime juice and keep aside.

5. Place the broccoli in the blender and puree smooth, add the remaining coconut milk (if any) or a little water to help the blades pick up the solids.

6. Return the broccoli mousse to the pan you cooked it in, season with salt and keep aside.

7. Heat an oven to 200 degrees (375 F).

8. Place the salmon prawn mix in greased moulds and bake in the oven for 10 to 12 minutes. They should feel firm and springy. Allow cooling for a few minutes and remove them from the moulds.

9. While the salmon is cooking remove the head and shell from the remaining prawns, leaving the tails on. Fry them in a small skillet until browned on both sides, about 1 minute.

10. To finish the dish, reheat the broccoli puree. Place a salmon tart on the centre of a plate, arrange some broccoli puree on the side, drizzle some papaya sauce around the tart and garnish with a fried prawn.

Nutritional values are manually calculated and based on the ingredients specified.
Nutritional value per serving: Calories: 608.9 Fat: 23.6g. Saturated Fat: 4.5g. Sodium: 1655.8mg. Carbohydrate 42.2g Protein: 52.9g. Dietary fibre: 5.4g.

HOT SMOKED SALMON WITH PICKLED VEGETABLES

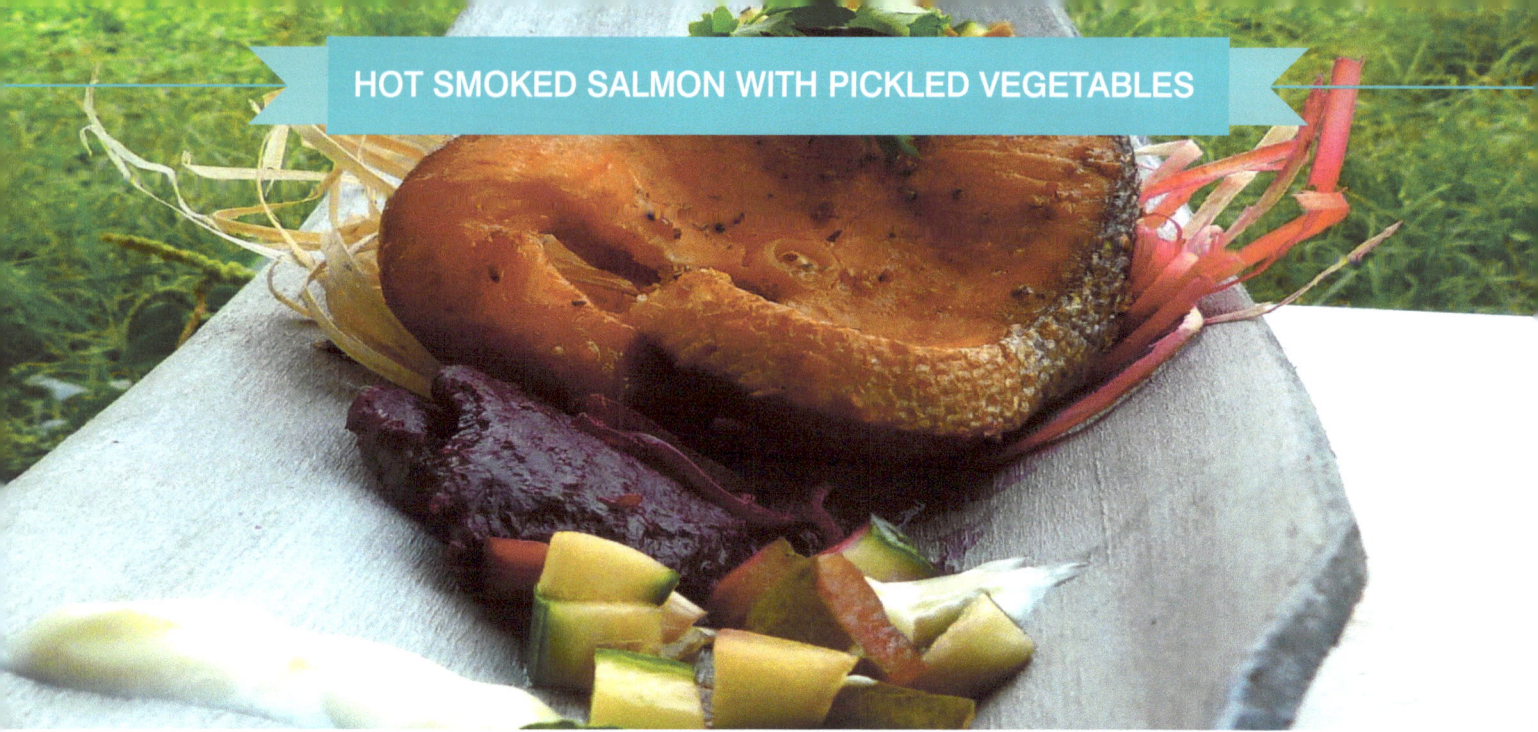

Preparation time: 20 mins

Cooking time: 10 mins

Total time: 30 mins

Hot smoked salmon is simply divine, but not always easily available, the good news is that it is very easy to make at home and a lot cheaper. Together with pickled vegetables and a Coyo dip, this dish makes a nice starter or light lunch.

Ingredients:

Serves 4

- 4 salmon steaks or salmon fillet (180gr, 6oz) each
- 2 sprigs rosemary
- 2 sprigs thyme • 125gr (½ cup) radish (sliced)
- 400 ml (1 ½ cup) water • 90 ml (3 tbsp) vinegar
- Wood chips • Sea salt

- 125gr (½ cup) cucumber cut in small cubes
- 60gr (2 tbsp) coconut sugar
- 15gr (1 tbsp) chopped dill
- 125gr (½ cup) beetroot (cooked and sliced small)
- 60gr (2 tbsp) red onion (sliced)

Method:

1. Place the vegetables individually over 3 containers; add the onions to the beetroot and the dill to the cucumber.
2. Bring the water, vinegar, sugar and a little salt to a boil, check for taste and divide over the three bowls. Allow cooling.
3. Use an old pan or skillet to smoke the salmon.
4. Line the base of the pan with a piece of aluminium foil. Add some wood chips; sprinkle with a bit of water.
5. Now you need something to elevate the salmon from the wood chips, if you have a small rack, great, if not a few (steel) cookie cutters will do the trick.
6. Season the salmon with a little salt, place them on the rack, cover the pan and turn on the heat until the chips start to smoke.
7. Lower the heat a bit, and smoke for 10 minutes.
8. Turn off the heat and allow cooling in the pan under cover.
9. When the salmon has cooled to room temperature, arrange the vegetable pickles over plates, top with the lukewarm salmon and serve with a dip of Coyo, salt and a squeeze of lemon.

Nutritional values are manually calculated and based on the ingredients specified.
Nutritional value per serving: Calories: 317.4 Fat: 12.8g Saturated Fat: 1.9g Sodium: 89.3mg. Sugar: 7.1g Carbohydrate 7.9g Protein: 40.3g Dietary fibre: 7.9g

JAPANESE MAKI ROLL WITH DAIKON

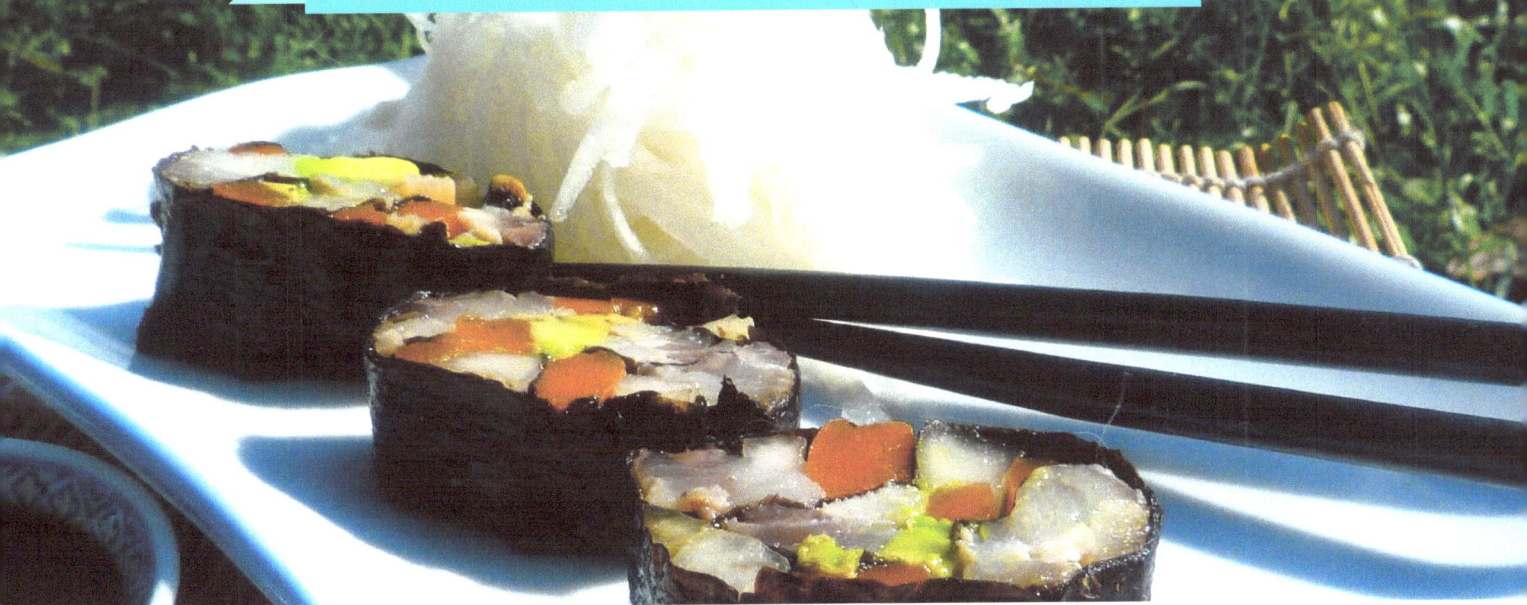

Preparation time:	Cooking time:	Marinating Time:	Total time:
15 minutes	05 minutes	1 hr	1hr 20 minutes

If you like Japanese food, going AIP will make you think Sushi is gone for good. Thankfully there is also maki. Check this lovely roll out, served with daikon (Japanese radish) and a coconut amino dip. The recipe has cured fish and pickled veggies rolled in seaweed sheets, divine!

Ingredients:

Serves 4

FOR THE VEGGIES:

- Carrot, radish, cucumber, avocado (90 gm, 3 tbsp each) cut into double sized match sticks
- 4 seaweed sheets
- 125ml (½ cup) lemon juice   •   Juice of 2 limes
- 60g (2 tbsp) maple syrup

- Sea salt, Water
- 450g (1 pound) shredded daikon or white radish

FOR THE FISH:

- 2 white fish fillets (180g, 6 oz each)
- Sea salt

Method:

1. Ensure the fish fillets are free of bones, place them on a tray and sprinkle with salt on both sides. Add the lime juice and rub it on both sides of the fillets. Marinade for at least an hour in the fridge.

2. You will see that the fish turns white on the outside, this means that the lime juice 'cooks' the fish, also called curing or cerviche.
3. Cook the carrot, radish and cucumber in equal parts of lemon juice, water and maple syrup over low heat until softened, but still a bit crunchy. Allow cooling.

4. Slice the fish crosswise in slices.
5. Place two sheets of the seaweed on a Japanese sushi mat so that you get a long sheet.
6. Arrange slices of fish, veggie and avocado on the bottom of the seaweed sheet. Roll and repeat until both sheets of seaweed are filled and rolled up.
7. Slice the roll in 1 cm (¾ inch) slices, arrange on plates and serve with the daikon and a dip of coconut amino.

Nutritional values are manually calculated and based on the ingredients specified.
Nutritional value per serving: Calories: 200.0 Fat: 4.9g Saturated Fat: 0.4g Sodium: 259.9 mg. Sugar: 10.7g Carbohydrate 20.5g Protein: 21.4g Dietary fibre: 3.4g

STEAMED WHITE FISH WITH CELERY, GINGER AND COCONUT BUTTER

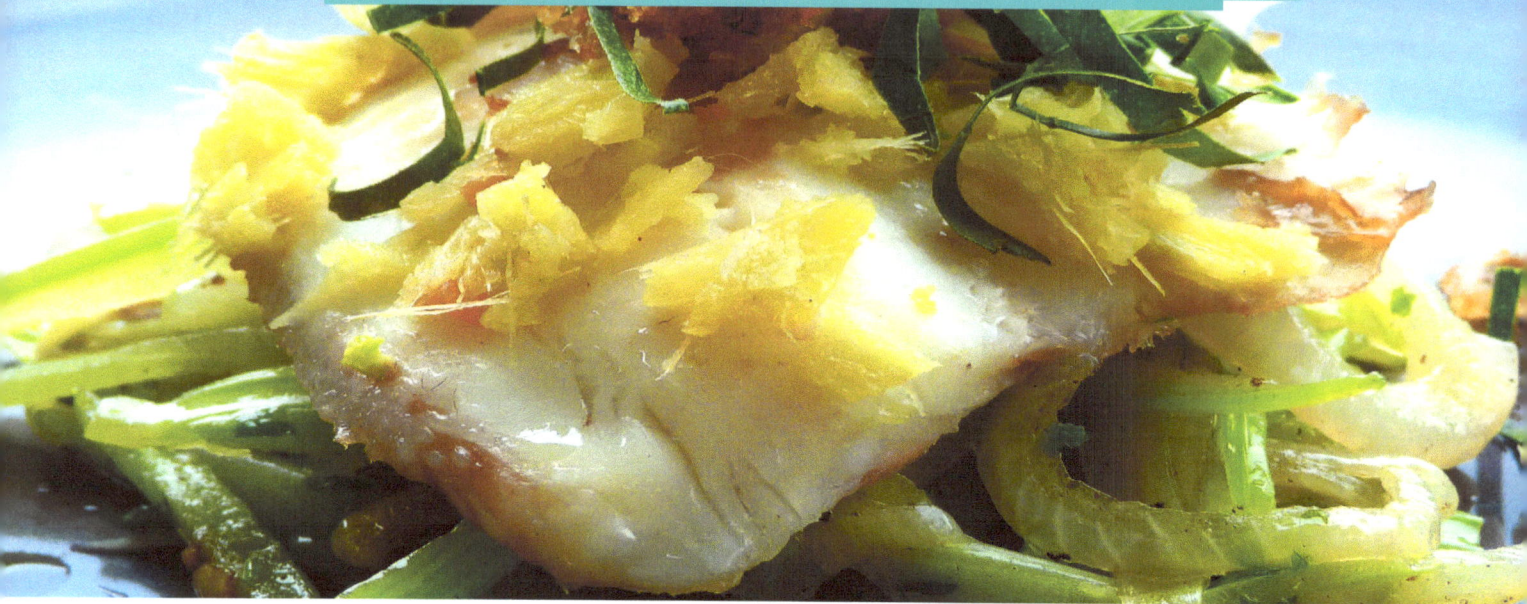

Preparation time: 25 minutes

Cooking time: 10 minutes

Marinating Time: 10 minutes

Total time: 45 minutes

The punchy Asian flavour in this dish really makes the fish sing. Steaming food is very healthy; the high heat of steam preserves the nutrients in the food because the process is quick, which also makes for a quick easy meal. Use any white fish you like.

Ingredients:

Serves 4

- 4 skinless white fish fillets (170gr, 6 oz) each
- 60g (2 tbsp) thinly sliced ginger
- 600g (1 ½ pound) celery (sliced in 8 cm, 3 inch long strips)
- Sea salt   • 2 cloves garlic (grated)   • 60ml (2 tbsp) olive oil
- 90g (3 tbsp) coconut butter A
- 20g (1 ½ tbsp) chopped parsley
- 1 medium onion (sliced in half moon pieces)

Method:

1. Prepare your steamer.
2. Place the fish fillets on a plate, rub with the ginger and let marinade for 10 minutes.
3. Meanwhile heat a skillet with the oil to medium high heat.
4. Place the fish with plate in your steamer and cover. Simultaneously add the onion, garlic, celery and parsley to the skillet.
5. Stir fry the vegetables for 2 to 3 minutes, season and drain out excess oil.
6. This will take about 3 to 4 minutes. Meanwhile your fish is also cooked.
7. Remove the fish from the steamer and allow to rest, remove the vegetables from the skillet and keep aside.
8. Add the coconut butter to the skillet and cook until slightly browned; you may need to add a little oil to the butter so it doesn't dry up too much.
9. Arrange some celery on plates, top with a fish fillet and drizzle some coconut butter around the dish.
10. Garnish with thinly sliced lime leaves.

Nutritional values are manually calculated and based on the ingredients specified.
Nutritional value per serving: Calories: 379.2. Fat: 20.0g Saturated Fat: 9.4g Sodium: 139.4mg. Sugar: 6.9g Carbohydrate 31.4g Protein: 20.4g Dietary fibre: 9.2g

WHITE GAZPACHO WITH CRAB AND PICKLED RADISH

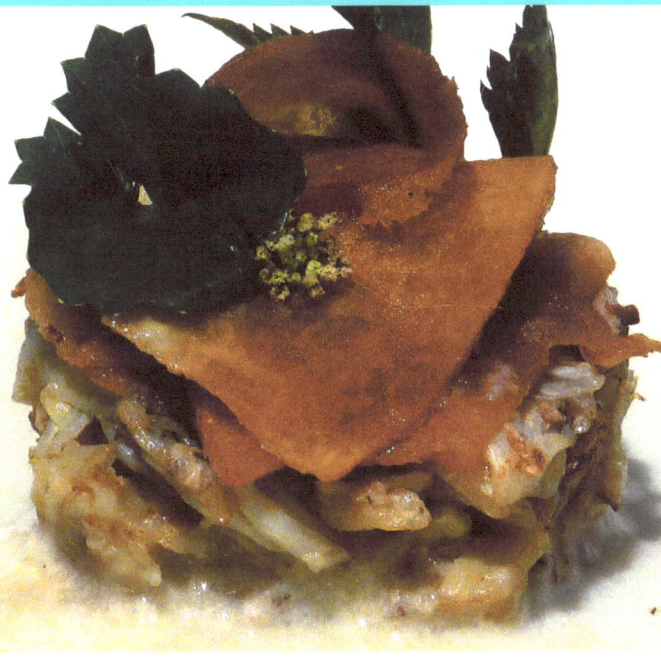

Preparation time: 20 mins

Cooking time: 10 mins

Total time: 30 mins

In the past there was nothing like a refreshing chilled bowl of Gazpacho on a hot summer's day...but what was I to do without my beloved nightshades? Be a little innovative! Gazpacho is a traditional Spanish soup; it is usually a combination of cucumber and tomato. Here horseradish replaces the tomato and the sweet crab balances the heat added. A little twist on this classic! Fresh sweet and sour pickled radish completes the dish.

Ingredients: Serves 4

FOR THE GAZPACHO:

- 600 ml (1 ½ pound) cucumber (peeled and de-seeded)
- 60gr (2 tbsp) grated horseradish
- 1 medium onion (cut small) • 2 cloves garlic (sliced)
- Sea salt • 25 ml (½ cup) coconut milk

FOR THE CRAB: • 200gr (6 ½ oz) cooked crabmeat

- 2 stalks chives (finely sliced) • 2 shallots (finely sliced)
- Sea salt   **FOR THE PICKLES:**
- 12 thin slices radish • 125ml (½ cup) water
- 60ml (2 tbsp) apple cider vinegar • Coconut sugar to taste

Method:

1. Start by making the pickles. Bring the water, vinegar and sugar to a boil, add the mix to the radish slices and allow to pickle for an hour or longer.
2. Cut the cucumber in small pieces and place with the horseradish, onion and garlic in an up-right blender. Blend smooth; add the coconut milk and pulse to combine.
3. Check for taste and strain through a fine sieve.
4. Combine the crabmeat with the shallot and chives, season with salt.
5. Place some crabmeat in the centre of a deep plate, pour gazpacho around it and garnish with the pickles.
6. Serve chilled.

Nutritional values are manually calculated and based on the ingredients specified.
Nutritional value per serving: Calories: 93.5. Fat: 1.8g Saturated Fat: 0.6g Sodium: 269.3 mg. Sugar: 9.3g Carbohydrate 11.7g Protein: 8.4g Dietary fibre: 1.1g

WOK FRIED MUD CRAB WITH SPRING ONION, GINGER AND GARLIC

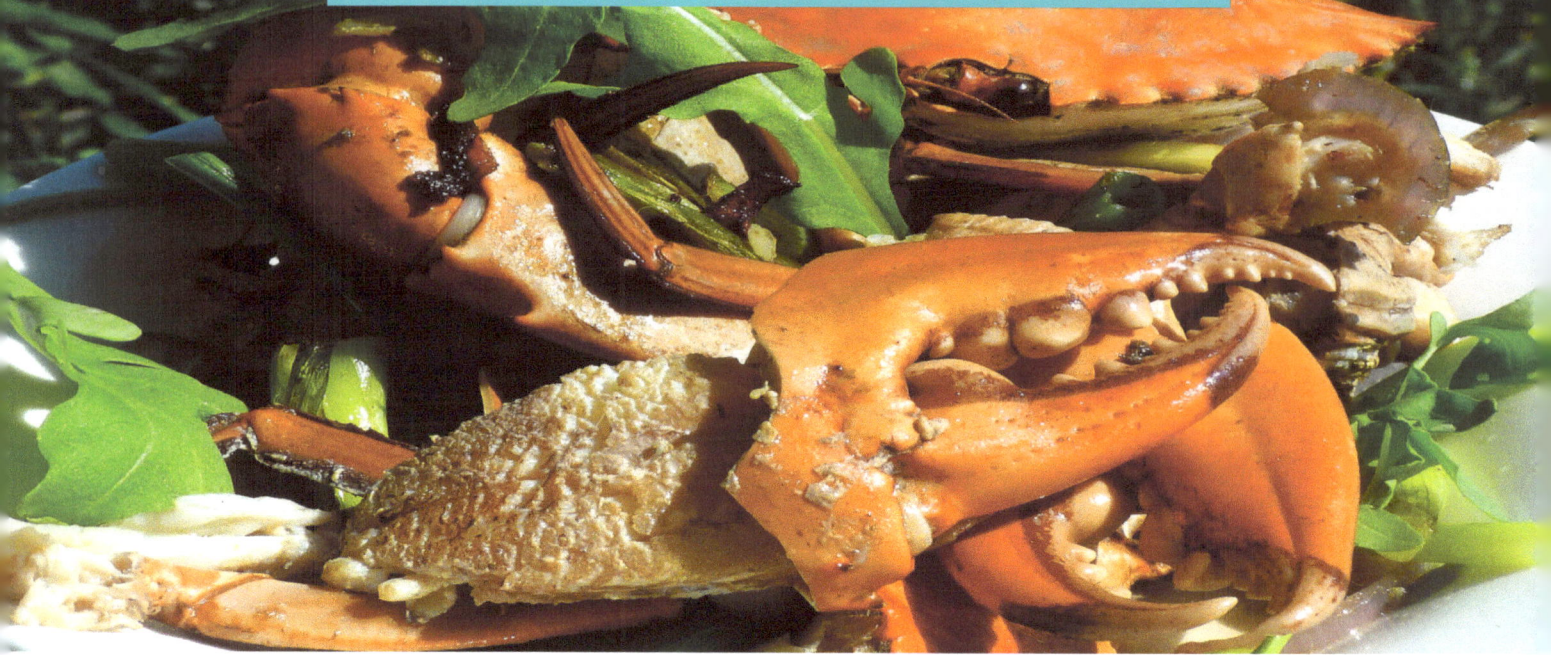

Preparation time: 15 mins

Cooking time: 10 mins

Total time: 25 mins

Nothing says Aussie summers to me like fresh mud crab! Eating crab, is eating crab, you need your hands and a bed sheet around your neck. There is not much else to it; it is crab all the way. Get sticky, get messy! Add other dishes to it if you like. Here is how to do the crab.

Ingredients:

Serves 4

- 4 mud crabs (500 to 600gr, 1 to 1.25 pounds) each
- 1 big red onion (roughly cut)
- 90 ml (3 tbsp) olive oil

- 2 cm (1 inch) piece ginger (sliced)
- 3 cloves garlic (sliced)
- 6 stalks spring onion (sliced)   • Pink salt

Method:

1. You need live crabs for this recipe. If you are not sure how to handle the crabs, ask your fishmonger to cut them in pieces for you.
2. Heat the oil in a heavy skillet to high heat; add the onions, ginger and garlic, and fry for 30 seconds.
3. Add the crab pieces and fry for 4 to 5 minutes, stirring them around every minute or so.
4. When the crab pieces change their colour to red, add ½ cup of bone broth, cover the pan and cook for 3 minutes.
5. Add the spring onion and combine.
6. Serve hot.

Nutritional values are manually calculated and based on the ingredients specified.
Nutritional value per serving: Calories: 107.2 Fat: 4.5g Saturated Fat: 0.6g Sodium: 159.7mg. Sugar: 0.0g Carbohydrate 4.4g Protein: 12.0g Dietary fibre: 0.8g

POULTRY

CHICKEN POT PIE WITH SPINACH CRUST

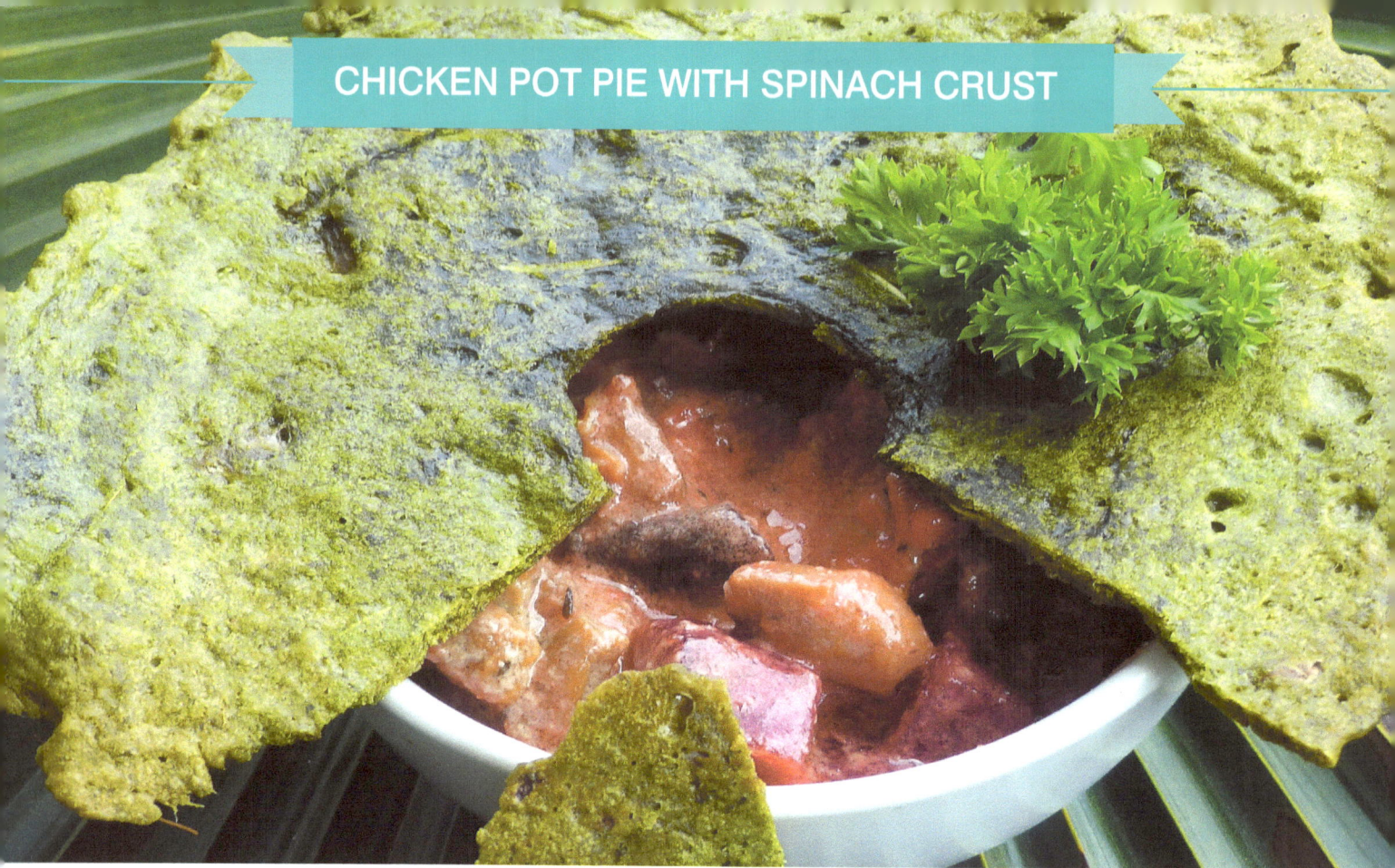

Preparation time: 15 mins

Cooking time: 30 mins

Total time: 45 mins

Chicken pot pie is something many people crave for, it is soul food. Without that crisp puff pastry on top the whole thing doesn't seem real anymore. Luckily there is another way to get a crisp finish to this popular dish. With a bit of effort you can get your crunchy pastry to dip into the creamy gravy!

Ingredients: Serves 4

FOR THE INSIDE:

- 600g (1 ½ pound) bone-less chicken thigh (cut into cubes)
- 1 medium onion (cut in half moon pieces)
- 1 medium sized carrot (cut in chunky pieces)
- 150g (5 oz) parsnip (sliced small) • 125ml (½ cup) chicken or bone broth

FOR THE CRUST:

- 250g (1cup) spinach pulp
- 180g (6 tbsp) tapioca starch
- 20g (1 tsp) onion powder • Pink salt

- 3 cloves garlic (chopped) • Pink salt
- 1 large stalk of celery (cut in chunky pieces)
- 150g (5 oz) beetroot (sliced small)
- 10g (1 tsp) thyme • 60ml (2 tbsp) olive oil
- 10g (1 tsp) sage • 125ml (½ cup) coconut cream

- 50g (1 ¾ tbsp) olive oil
- 10g (1 tsp) baking soda
- 20g (1 tsp) garlic powder

Method:

1. Heat the oil in a skillet to medium heat; add the onion and garlic, fry for 1 minute.

2. Add the chicken plus the thyme, sage and a little salt, fry until the chicken has browned.

3. Add all the vegetables and fry for another 2 minutes.

4. Add the broth, lower the heat and simmer for 10 minutes.

5. Add the coconut cream and bring to a boil, check for taste and remove from the heat.

6. Divide the mix over 4 oven proof baking dishes.

7. Meanwhile heat an oven to 200 degrees (375 F).

8. Combine the spinach pulp (if you don't have any, boil spinach, drain and blend smooth) with the other ingredients until a soft dough forms.

9. Brush a sheet of aluminium foil with some oil and spread some of the dough on the sheet.

10. Make 4 rounds, about 2 cm (¾ inch) broader than your baking dishes, and 3 mm (1/8 inch) thickness.

11. Spreading the dough with wet fingers works well.

12. Cover the dough with another greased sheet and bake for 10 to 15 minutes in the oven.

13. Remove the crusts from the oven and cut a little hole in the centre of each one.

14. Place the crust sheets on top of each baking dish with pot pie mix, cover with aluminium foil and bake for another 15 minutes.

15. Serve hot.

Nutritional values are manually calculated and based on the ingredients specified.
Nutritional value per serving: Calories: 596.9. Fat: 24.2.0g. Saturated Fat: 5.9g. Sodium: 323.8mg. Sugar: 8.3g Carbohydrate 63.1g. Protein: 36.7g. Dietary fibre: 5.7g.

CHICKEN IN THE BASKET

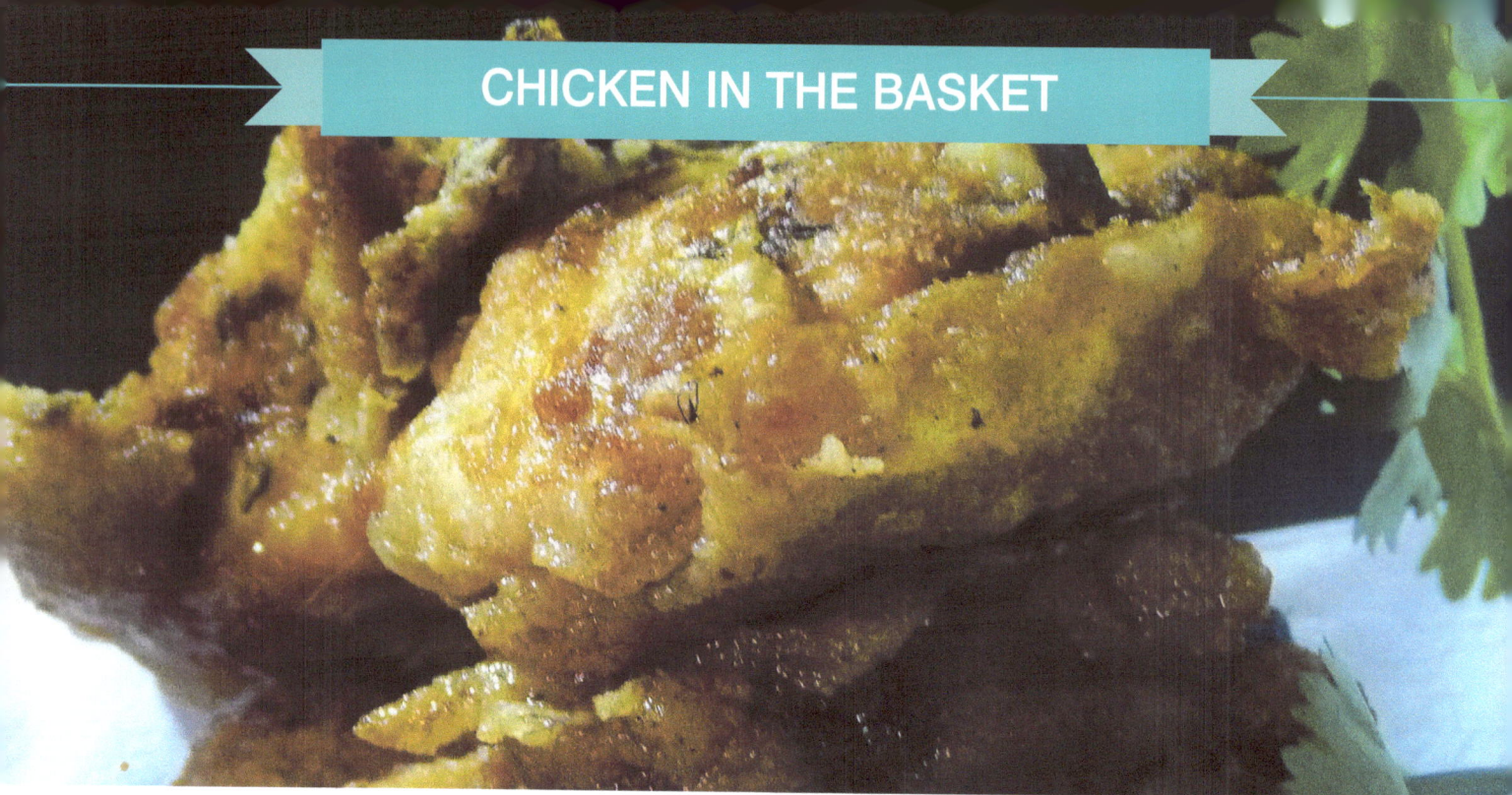

Preparation time: 15 mins

Cooking time: 25 mins

Total time: 40 mins

Who doesn't love crispy fried chicken!? Finger licking good but it is actually really good for you! The cooking method may not sound like fried at first, but you will get the best crispy fried chicken you have ever had.

Ingredients:

Serves 4

FOR THE CHICKEN:

- 1.6kg (4 pound) boneless, (skin on) chicken pieces
- 250gr (1 cup) tapioca flour
- 30gr (1 tbsp) dried sage
- 15gr (½ tbsp) garlic powder

- 250 ml (1 cup) palm oil
- Sea salt
- 15gr (½ tbsp) onion powder
- 30gr (1 tbsp) dried basil leaves
- 30gr (1 tbsp) dried oregano

Method:

1. Combine the tapioca flour with all of the herbs, onion, garlic and salt.
2. Heat the oil in a skillet to 160 degrees(320 F).
3. Coat the chicken pieces with the flour mix, ensure they are fully coated.
4. Place the chicken with some space in between them in the oil, don't touch or move them around. Fry for 10 minutes on one side, flip them over and fry another 10 minutes. You may have to do this in batches.
5. Transfer the chicken to an oven tray and finish in a pre-heated oven of 180 degrees (350 F) for another 5 minutes.
6. Serve hot.

Nutritional values are manually calculated and based on the ingredients specified.
Nutritional value per serving: Calories: 1206.7 Fat: 87.0g Saturated Fat: 19.0g Sodium: 0.7mg. Sugar: 0.2g Carbohydrate 28.9g Protein: 73.9g Dietary fibre: 1.9g

CHICKEN STIR FRY WITH MUSTARD LEAVES

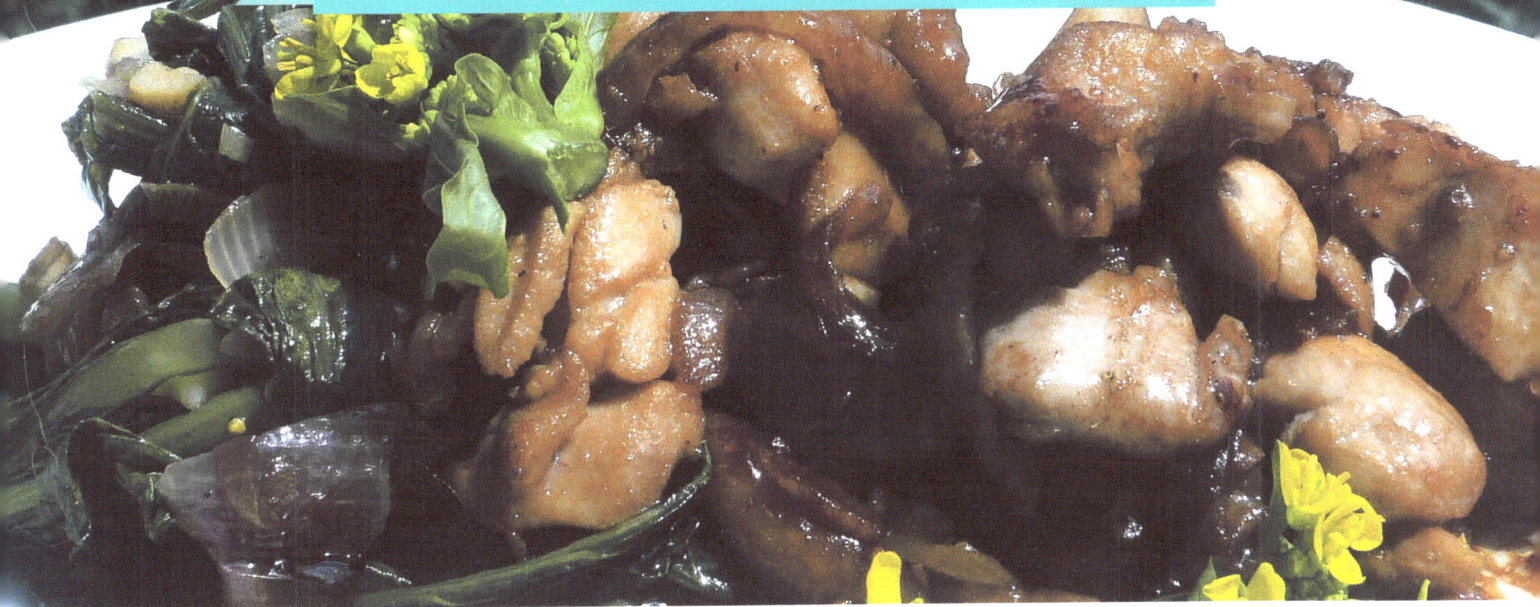

Preparation time: 20 mins

Cooking time: 10 mins

Marinating Time: 1 hr

Total time: 1.5 hr

A stir fry is easy, quick to make, tasty and healthy. About everything you look for in a dish. This is sure to be a family favourite! It ticks all the nutritional boxes and is so tasty!

Ingredients:

Serves 4

- 600g (1 ½ pound) Free range boneless (skin-on) chicken thighs
- 1 ½ medium size red onion (finely chopped)
- 2 ½ cm (1inch) piece of young ginger (grated)
- 2 cloves garlic (chopped)
- 60g (2 tbsp) coconut amino
- 600g (1 ½ pound) baby mustard leaves
- 120ml (4 tbsp) olive oil
- Pink salt

Method:

1. Slice the chicken thighs in 1 cm (1/2 inch) broad strips and place them in a bowl. Add the coconut amino, 2/3 of the onion and garlic, the ginger and combine. Allow to marinate for an hour.
2. Meanwhile remove the base of the mustard leaves and cut them in bite size pieces.
3. Heat half of the oil in a skillet; add the remainder of the onion followed by the mustard leaves. Stir fry the vegetables, stirring them regularly for 4 to 5 minutes. The vegetables should have softened by now but still have a crunchy texture. If this is not the case add a little water to the pan, which will steam them through.
4. Remove the vegetables from the pan and keep warm in a covered bowl.
5. Add the remaining olive oil to the pan and let it become smoking hot, add the chicken and stir fry, scoop them constantly around, they should be cooked and brown in 3 to 4 minutes.
6. Divide the mustard leaves over plates and top with the chicken strips.
7. Serve hot.

Nutritional values are manually calculated and based on the ingredients specified.
Nutritional value per serving: Calories: 333.8 Fat: 19.5g. Saturated Fat: 3.4g. Sodium: 195.3mg. Carbohydrate 7.3g Protein: 32.1g. Dietary fibre: 1.0g.

COCONUT COATED CHICKEN STRIPS
WITH COYO DIP

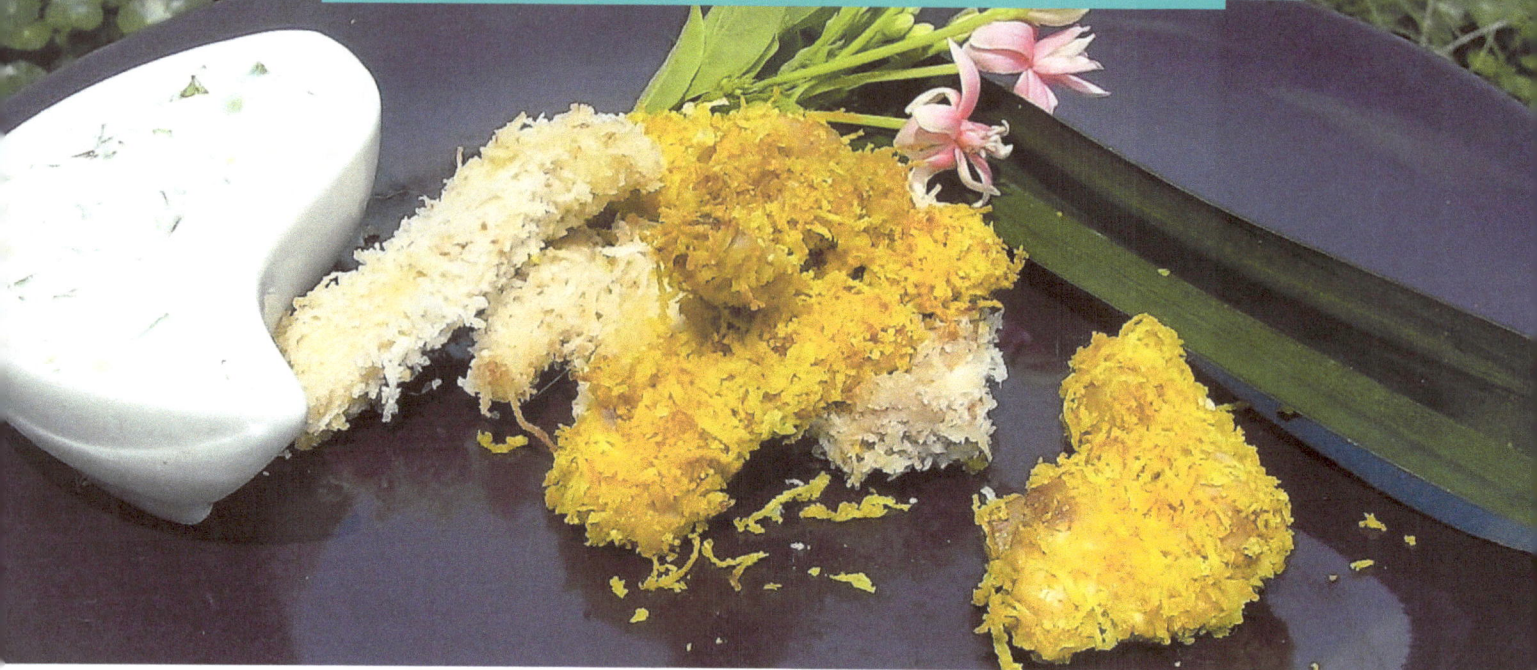

Preparation time: 15 mins

Cooking time: 15 mins

Total time: 30 mins

Succulent chicken leg meat with a crisp finish served with a refreshing dip. Be adventurous and add some ground ginger or chopped coriander!

Ingredients:

Serves 4

FOR THE CHICKEN:

- 500gr (1 pound) boneless chicken leg meat (cut into 1 ½ cm (½ inch) broad strips)
- 125gr (½ cup) coconut milk
- Pink salt
- 250gr (1 cup) shredded coconut
- ½ tsp turmeric powder (optional)

FOR THE COYO DIP:

- Salt
- 15gr (1 tbsp) chopped mint leaves
- 250ml (1 cup) coyo yoghurt
- 2 cloves garlic (minced)
- 60gr (2 tbsp) cucumber (deseeded and cut in small cubes)

Method:

1. Pre-heat an oven to 180 degrees (325 F).
2. Season the chicken strips with salt.
3. Turmeric gives a lovely colour after baking, if you decide to use it mix the turmeric with the shredded coconut or do half/ half for two different colours.
4. Dip the chicken strips in the coconut milk, roll them in the shredded coconut and place on a baking tray. The best way is to dip and coat the strips one by one, or it becomes a messy affair.
5. Bake the strips for 10 to 12 minutes in the oven turning them half way.
6. While the strips are baking, combine the dip ingredients.
7. Serve the strips with the dip on the side.

Nutritional values are manually calculated and based on the ingredients specified.
Nutritional value per serving: Calories: 259.8. Fat: 19.8g Saturated Fat: 1.3g Sodium: 63.1mg Carbohydrate 10.6g Protein: 15.2g Dietary fibre: 1.1g

CRACKLING CHICKEN THIGHS WITH COCONUT SPINACH AND CARROT

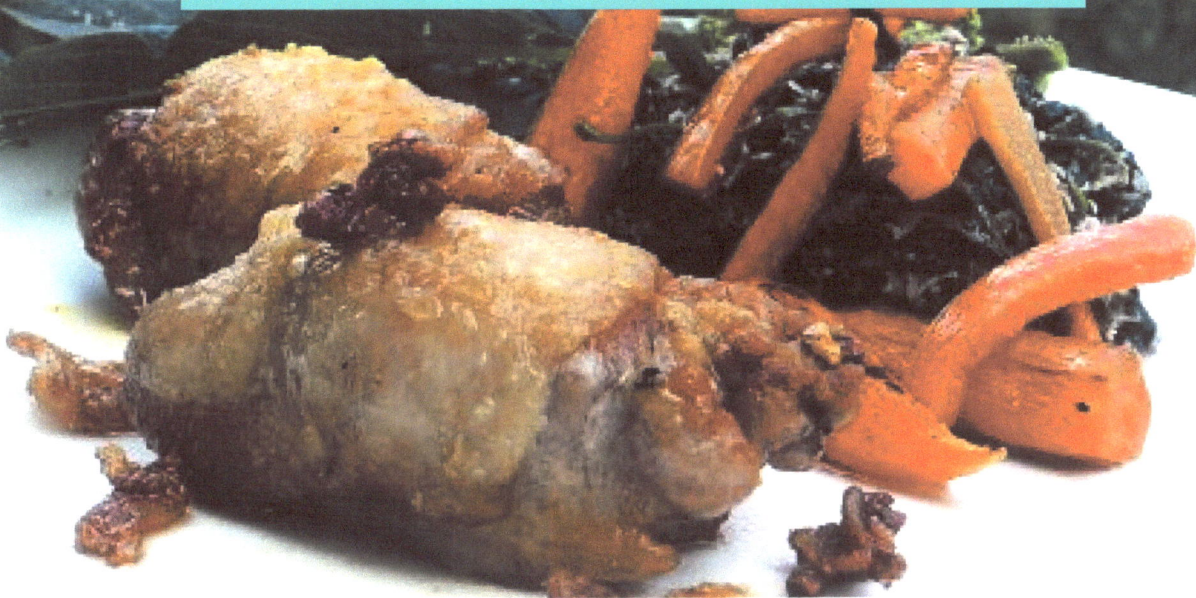

Preparation time: 20 mins

Cooking time: 15 mins

Total time: 35 mins

The four C's in the name of this recipe will stick in your mind! It truly is a dish to remember that you will want to cook over and over! Crackling is known for pork, but it works really well for chicken also. The crunchy, juicy chicken thighs and loads of veggies make this recipe a feast.

Ingredients: Serves 4

FOR THE CHICKEN THIGHS:

- 8 boneless (skin-on) chicken thighs
- 45g (1 ½ tbsp.) coarse Pink salt

FOR THE VEGGIES:

- 2 cloves garlic (chopped)

- 1 kg (2 ½ pounds) raw spinach
- 30g (1 tbsp olive oil) • 1 medium onion (cut in half moon rings)
- 1 ½ medium carrots cut into sticks
- 60g (3 tbsp) grated coconut • 90g (3 tbsp) raw chicken fat
- 125g (1/2 cup) coconut cream

Method:

1. Rub the salt on the skin of the chicken thighs.
2. Melt the chicken fat on medium heat. When melted turn the heat to high and fry the chicken thighs skin down on medium high heat, for 5 to 6 minutes in the chicken fat. The skin will release most of its fat during the process and turn golden and crunchy.
3. Turn the thighs and fry for another 2 to 3 minutes so they are cooked through.
4. Drain the thighs on a wire rack. Strain the fat through a sieve and reserve for later use. You will now have some crispy bits in the sieve, keep them aside.
5. Blanch the carrot sticks for 2 to 3 minutes, they should soften but still have crunch.
6. Heat the olive oil in a skillet, add the onions and garlic, fry for 1 minute, add the spinach and fry until wilted and soft about 5 minutes. If needed add a little water to prevent burning.
7. Drain the spinach in a colander and return to the pan. Add the fat bits and mix through. Add the coconut cream and shredded coconut, place the carrots on top, season with salt and simmer for another 5 minutes.
8. Divide the veggies over plates and top with the crackling chicken thighs.
9. Serve hot.

Nutritional values are manually calculated and based on the ingredients specified.
Nutritional value per serving: Calories: 719.2. Fat: 58.3g Saturated Fat: 15.7g Sodium: 2984.1mg Carbohydrate 16.0g Protein: 35.0g Dietary fibre: 15.3g

CRISPY DUCK LEG WITH COLESLAW

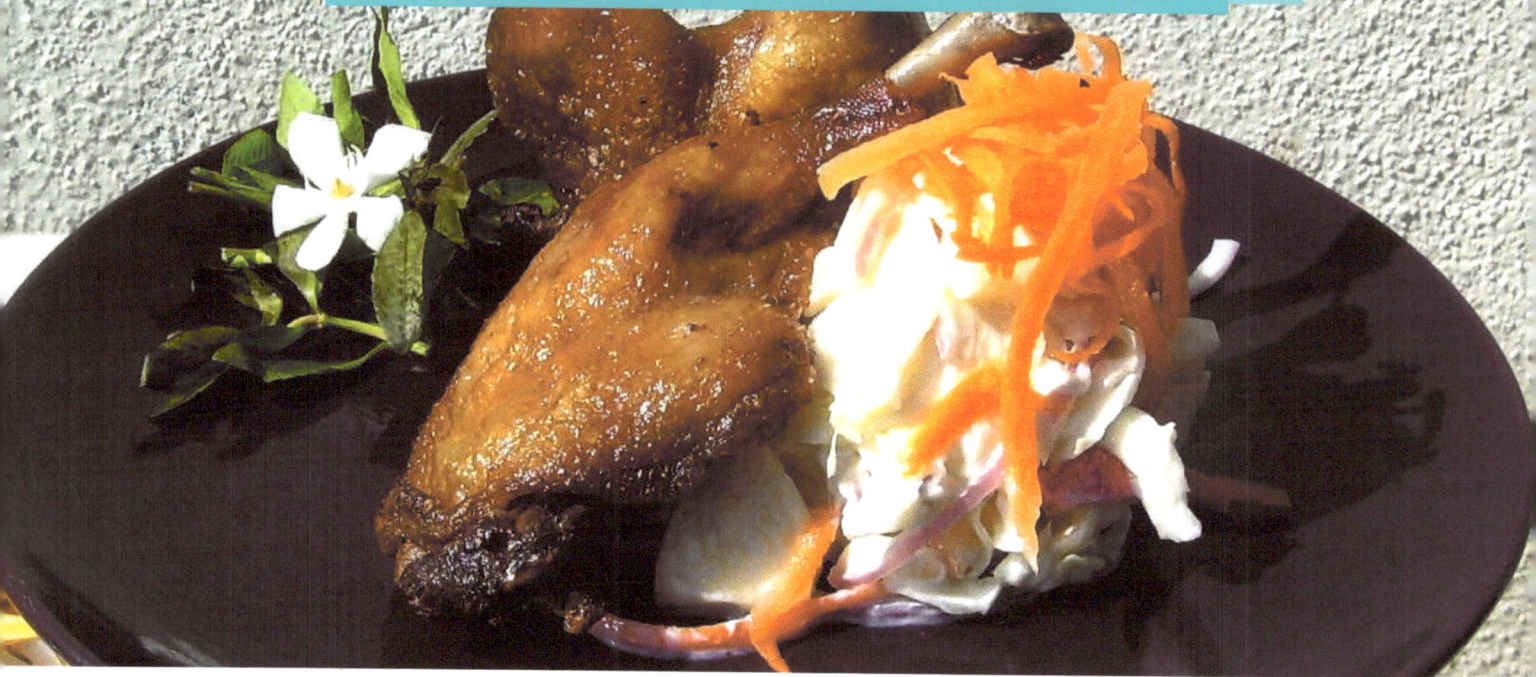

Preparation time:
20 mins

Cooking time:
1hr 30 mins

Total time:
1 hr 50 mins

Nothing can make my mouth water faster than when I think about eating duck with duck fat. I absolutely love it and it is so good for you. Duck fat has a high smoke point, this means you can cook with it at very hot temperatures without it smoking or adopting an off flavour. Unlike butter or olive oil, duck fat can be recycled. The greatest of all is the rich taste and flavour. This amazing AIP dish will impress your friends and have them asking you for the recipe, you better cook more so they can take some home!

Ingredients:

Serves 4

FOR THE DUCK LEG:

* 8pcs of duck leg (skin on and with leg bones)

* 250gr (1 cup) duck fat
* Pink salt

FOR THE COLESLAW:

* 300gr (10 oz) shredded white cabbage
* 1 medium sized red onion (chopped)

* 150gr (5 oz) shredded carrot

* 1 hard green apple (Granny Smith) peeled, cored and sliced in small piecess

* 60ml (2 tbsp) lemon juice

* 125gr (1/2 cup) yoghurt dressing

* 30gr (2 tbsp) fresh cilantro (chopped)

Method:

1. Pre- heat an oven to 125 degrees (257 F).
2. Melt the duck fat in a Dutch oven and add the duck legs, cover the pan with a lid and place in the oven.
3. Cook the duck legs completely soft in the fat, this may take 1 ½ hours. Test by piercing a small knife through the meat and twist, if the meat is fork tender, remove the pan from the oven, transfer the legs to a tray and allow cooling in the fridge, preferably overnight. Reserve the duck fat.
4. Combine the salad ingredients in a mixing bowl and combine, check for taste.
5. Heat the duck fat to 180 degrees (325 F), add the duck legs and fry them crispy and golden in 3 to 4 minutes.
6. Serve hot with a serving of coleslaw on the side.

Nutritional values are manually calculated and based on the ingredients specified.
Nutritional value per serving: Calories: 771.4 Fat: 46.4g. Saturated Fat: 11.8g. Sodium: 727.9mg Carbohydrate 17.4g. Protein: 70.0g. Dietary fibre: 4.2g.

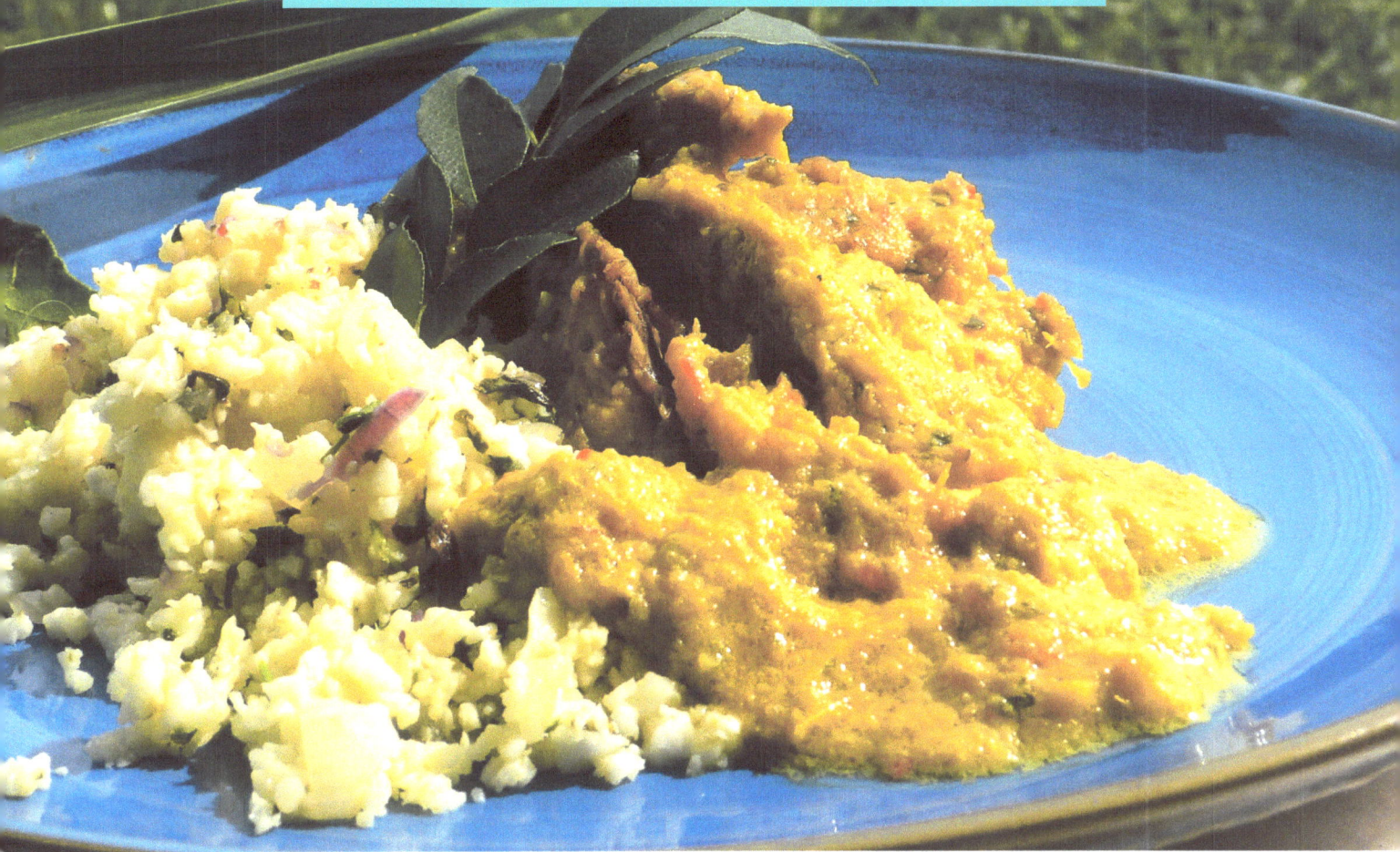

Preparation time: 20 mins

Cooking time: 30 mins

Total time: 50 mins

Asian curries are very flavoursome, even without the chilli, which is unwavering in these dishes. Without rice they seem a bit messy to eat, but cauliflower rice is a good substitute. Be adventurous with your cauli rice and add aromatics such as citrus zest, shredded coconut or a pinch or two of turmeric, ginger or garlic powder. Or another different combo e.g. half broccoli and half cauliflower rice.

Ingredients:

Serves 4

FOR THE CURRY:

- 1200g (3 pounds) free range, bone–in chicken pieces (chicken thighs or drumsticks are fine)

- 2 red onions (roughly chopped)

- 3 cloves garlic • 20g (1/2 tbsp) turmeric powder

- 1 stalk lemongrass • 2 ½ cm (1 inch) piece of young ginger root

- 4 Kaffir lime leaves (optional)

- 10 curry leaves (optional)

- 1 cinnamon stick • 60ml (2 tbsp palm oil)

- 250ml (1 cup) coconut milk • Pink salt

FOR THE CAULIFLOWER RICE:

- 600g (1 ½ pound) cauliflower florets

- 60g (2 tbsp) olive oil

- Pink salt to taste

Method:

(1) Ask your butcher to cut the chicken in small pieces. The size should be similar to a half a drumstick.

(2) Heat the palm oil in a skillet, season the chicken pieces with salt and brown them all around, remove from the pan and keep aside.

(3) Lime and curry leaves are not always available, if you have them remove the centre stalk from the lime and remove the curry leaves from the stalk they grow on.

(4) Remove the woody leaves from the lemon grass, remove the base and slice the white part, discard the top green part. If your knife doesn't go through the leaves anymore you have reached the end.

(5) Place all other ingredients except for the coconut milk in an up-right blender, add a little water so the blades pick-up the solids and blend into a paste.

(6) Re-heat the oil still in the pan; add the paste and cinnamon stick and fry until fragrant, 3 to 4 minutes.

(7) Add the chicken and mix through.

(8) Add the coconut milk and bring to a slow boil, boiling too fast may curdle the coconut milk.

(9) When the curry cooks, cover the pan and continue cooking for about 20 minutes until the chicken is tender.

(10) Meanwhile place the cauliflower in a food processor and pulse until you have a rice like texture, scraping the sides of the bowl along the way.

(11) Heat the olive oil in a skillet; add the onions followed by the cauliflower rice. Fry for 2 to 3 minutes until the cauliflower softens, but still has a crunch, season with salt.

(12) Place the curry and cauliflower rice in different serving trays and serve.

**Nutritional values are manually calculated and based on the ingredients specified.
Nutritional value per serving: Calories:** 771.4 Fat: 46.4g. Saturated Fat: 11.8g. Sodium: 727.9mg Carbohydrate 17.4g. Protein: 70.0g. Dietary fibre: 4.2g.

FRIED CHICKEN BREAST IN BROTH

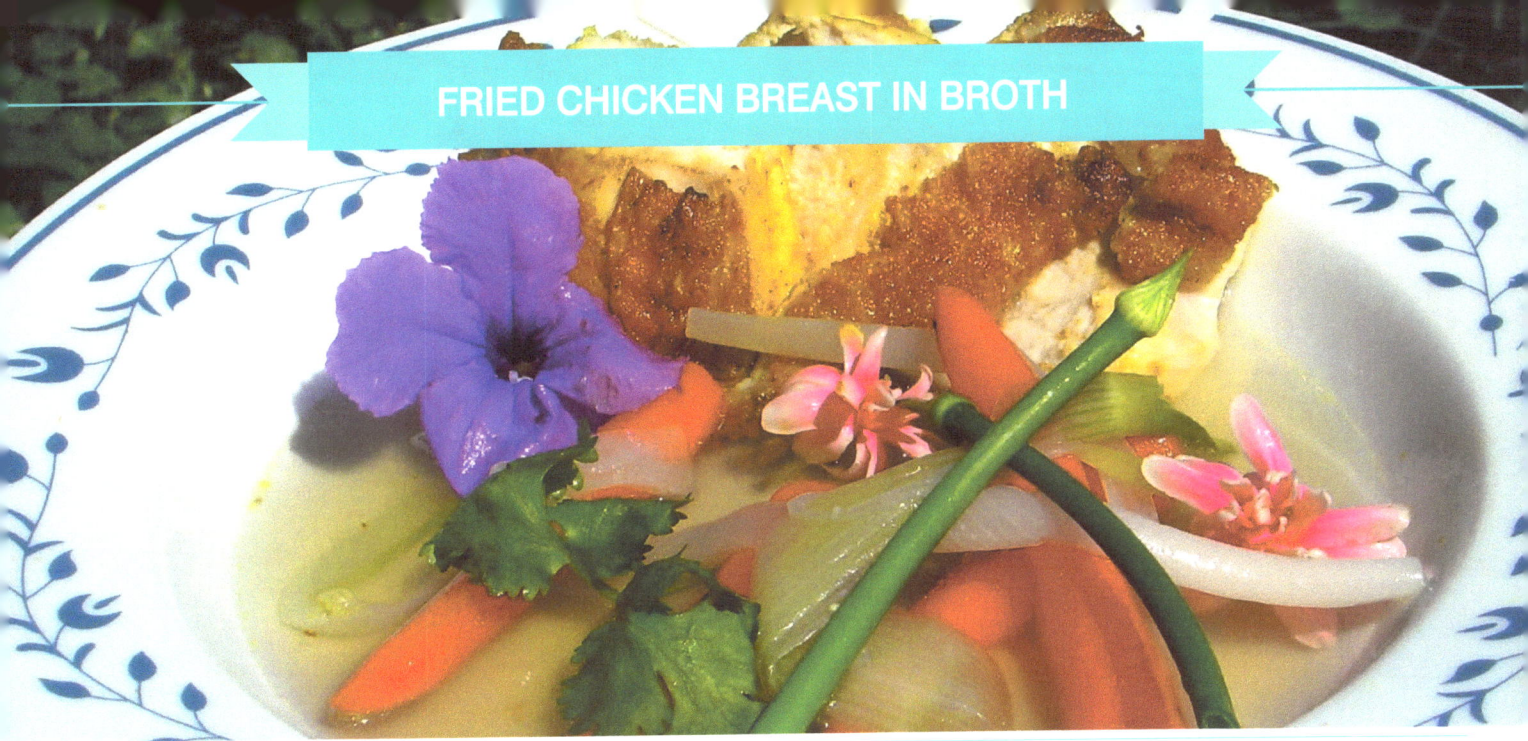

Preparation time: 10 mins

Cooking time: 15 mins

Total time: 25 mins

A good strong broth is known to have a multitude of beneficial health properties, like collagen, minerals, gelatin and a complete amino acid profile. Drinking broth by itself is so healing for your gut, and turning it into a meal is even better.

Ingredients:

Serves 4

- 600g (1 ¼ lbs) skin-on free range chicken breast
- 30g (1 tbsp) turmeric powder
- 4 sprigs of organic thyme
- 300g (10 oz) organic baby carrots
- 300g (10 oz) organic leek (cut in 10 cm, 2 ½ inch strips)
- 750ml (3 cups) bone broth
- Few coriander leaves for garnish
- Salt
- 90g (3 tbsp) olive oil

Method:

1. Pre-heat an oven to 180 degrees (325 F).
2. Make a small incision length wise on the thick side of the chicken fillet. Place a sprig of thyme in each pocket. Season with salt and rub the turmeric powder all over the fillets.
3. Heat the oil in a skillet to medium heat. Add the chicken breast, skin down first and fry golden brown in 3 to 4 minutes. Flip them over, transfer to the oven and finish baking for 10 to 12 minutes. When the fillets feel firm and bouncy if you press on them, they are cooked through. Remove the thyme and allow resting while finishing the broth.
4. Bring the broth to a boil and lower the heat. Add the carrots and simmer for 5 to 7 minutes or until the carrots are soft, but still a bit crunchy.
5. Add the leeks about 1 minute before serving.
6. Place the broth and vegetables in serving bowls or plates, slice the chicken fillets and add to the broth.
7. Garnish with coriander leaves.

Nutritional values are manually calculated and based on the ingredients specified.
Nutritional value per serving: Calories: 407.7 Fat: 21.5g Saturated Fat: 5.6g Sodium: 88.1mg. Carbohydrate 19.6g Protein: 34.0g Dietary fibre: 3.8g

GRILLED CHICKEN BREAST WITH ROASTED BROCCOLI AND SWEET POTATO MASH

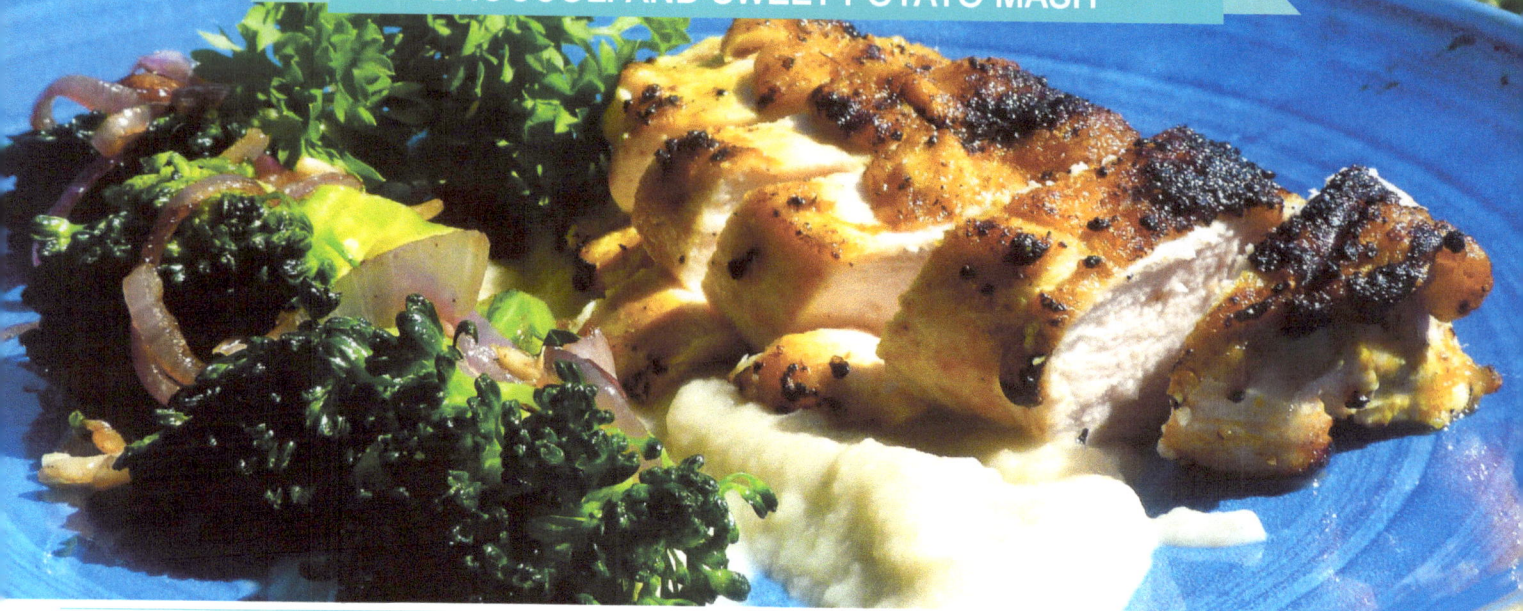

Preparation time: 20 mins

Cooking time: 25 mins

Total time: 45 mins

This is a perfect dish for any day of the week; quick and flavoursome and it will also work well with chicken thighs. This is great as a freeze ahead dish too. Just double the quantity of chicken and portion into zip lock bags. When you have a busy week just defrost the chicken in the fridge, and you have the protein ready to serve with a simple salad or steamed veggies!

Ingredients: Serves 4

- 4 skin-on chicken breast (approx. 170gm (6 oz) each
- 30g (3 tsp) turmeric powder
- 30g (3tsp) ground ginger
- 30g (3tsp) garlic powder • Zest of a lemon or lime
- 1/2 tbsp dried mint

- 900g (2 pounds) sweet potatoes (cut into pieces)
- 60g (2 tbsp) chopped onion • 30g (2 tsp) chopped garlic
- 125ml (½ cup) coconut milk
- 90ml (3 tbsp) olive oil • Pink salt
- Lime or lemon wedges • 600g (1 ½ pound) broccoli floets

Method:

1. Boil about 1 litre of water in a pot with a little salt. Add the broccoli florets when the water boils and blanch for two minutes. Drain and cool in iced water.
2. Season the chicken breast with salt, turmeric, ginger and garlic powder, mint and zest and 2/3 of the oil.
   Boil the sweet potatoes with the onion and garlic until soft, 15 minutes, drain and mash.
3. Add the coconut milk and mix into a smooth mash.
4. Pre-heat an oven to 180 degrees (325 F). Combine the broccoli with the leftover oil and a little salt. Roast for 8 to 10 minutes in the oven.
5. Heat a grill or griddle to high heat, place the chicken breast skin down on the grill, and grill for 3 to 4 minutes. Turn them around and grill for another 2 to 3 minutes.
6. Arrange some mash on plates, top with the broccoli and lastly the grilled chicken breast and lime wedges.

Nutritional values are manually calculated and based on the ingredients specified.
Nutritional value per serving: Calories: 583.5. Fat: 27.5g Saturated Fat: 6.7g Sodium: 169.5mg. Sugar: 0.8g Carbohydrate 43.1g Protein: 42.5g Dietary fibre: 8.9g

GRILLED CHICKEN WINGS WITH RUSTIC SALAD

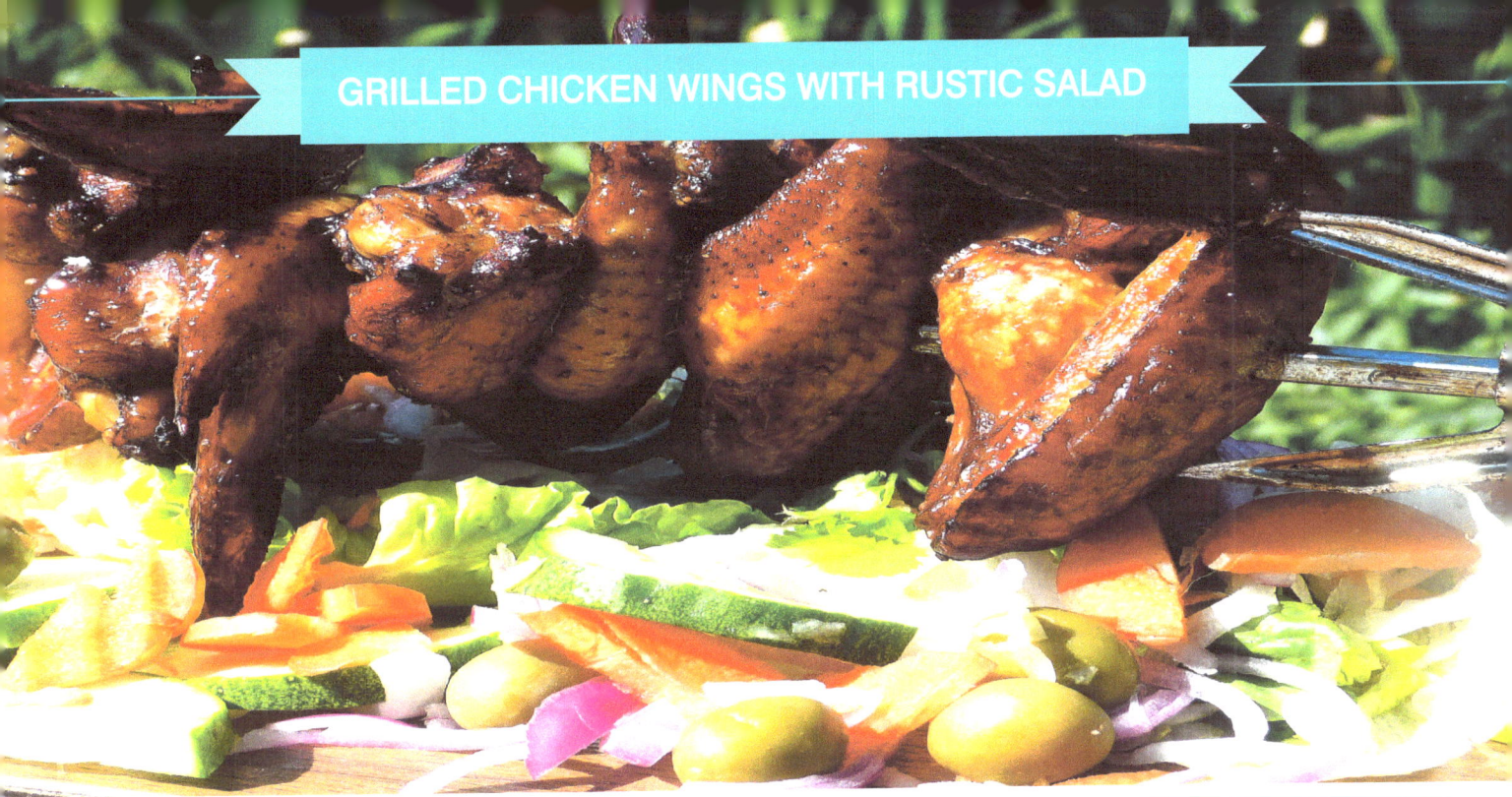

Preparation time: 15 mins

Cooking time: 30 mins

Marinating time: 3 hrs (or overnight)

Total time: 3 hrs 45 mins

Who doesn't love sticky chicken wings? Grilled with crispy edges and juicy meat, they are indeed irresistible, not to mention economical. I will often double this dish and freeze half into a zip lock bag for later use. Combined with a salad full of goodies, this is a dish to die for!

Ingredients: Serves 4

FOR THE CHICKEN WINGS:

- 16 chicken wings
- 125 ml (½ cup) coconut aminos
- 1 small onion (finely minced)
- 60ml (2 tbsp) olive oil
- ½ tbsp finely minced fresh ginger
- Pink salt, (if needed)
- 1tbsp apple cider vinegar

- 3 cloves garlic (grated)
- Raw honey to taste (optional)
- 3½ tbsp finely minced fresh turmeric

FOR THE SALAD:

- Any salad you like
- Sea salt
- Olive oil
- Any filling you like (carrot, radish, olives, capers, chopped fried bacon, zucchini, and anchovies)

Method:

1. Combine the coconut amino with the other ingredients, taste for the right balance of salty, sweet and sour. Add the chicken wings and marinate for a few hours or overnight.
2. If you use the Barbie, fry the wings until golden and crisp, 10 to 15 minutes. If you use an oven, cook them on the spit and grill for 20 minutes.
3. Meanwhile prepare the salad by mixing all ingredients you like and spread them over a serving board.
4. Top with the wings and serve with a dip of your choice.

Nutritional values are manually calculated and based on the ingredients specified.
Nutritional value per serving: Calories: 570.1. Fat: 38.4g. Saturated Fat: 8.6g. Sodium: 1554.1 mg. Sugar: 1.5g. Carbohydrate 29.8g Protein: 28.0g. Dietary fibre: 3.8 g.

ROASTED DUCK BREAST WITH LAVENDER, BEETROOT AND SWEET POTATO

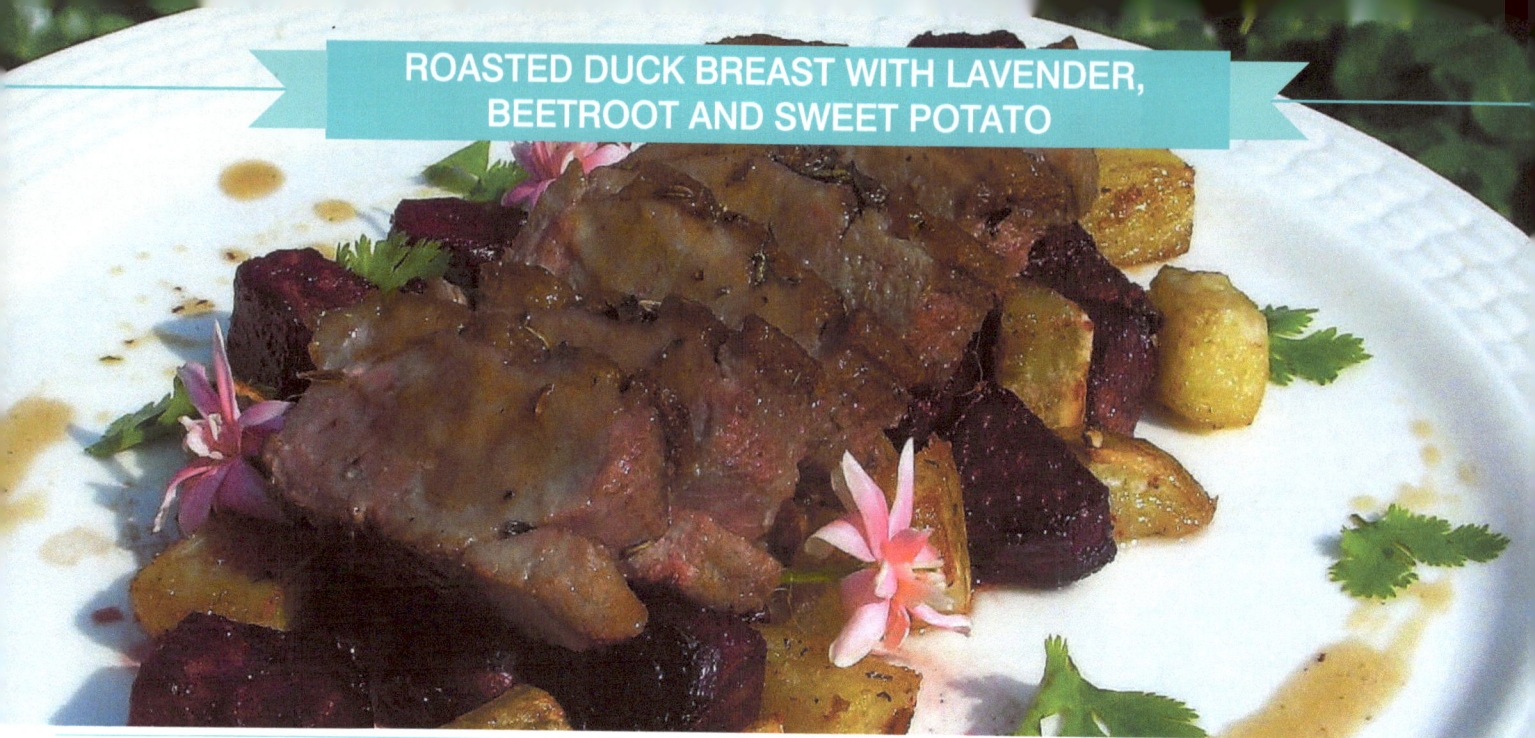

Preparation time: 15 mins

Cooking time: 50 mins

Total time: 65 mins

Spectacular may be an underrated word for this dish! Duck is one of my favourite game meats, there is nothing like crispy duck skin and perfectly pink duck meat...just heavenly! The diverse flavours of beetroot and sweet potatoes combined with lavender and a little sweetness from the maple syrup makes this a most surprising dish!

Ingredients: Serves 4

FOR THE DUCK BREAST:

* 4 bone-less (skin-on) duck breast

* 100ml (3 ¼ tbsp) maple syrup

* 10g (¾ tsp) tarragon • 15g (½ tbsp.) coarse pink salt

* 1/2 tbsp dried mint • 10g (¾ tsp) dry lavender

* 10g (¾ tsp thyme) • 30ml (1 tbsp) olive oil

FOR THE VEGGIES:

* 2 medium sized sweet potatoes (Hawaiian sweet potato works well)

* 6 small beetroots • 60 ml (2 tbsp) coconut butter

* 60 ml (2 tbsp) olive oil

Method:

1. Pre-heat an oven to 190 degrees (350 F).
2. Season the duck breasts with salt.
3. Cut the beetroot and sweet potatoes into large cubes, about 2 cm (1 inch square). Spread the beetroot and sweet potato cubes on a baking tray, sprinkle with a little salt and the olive oil and combine. Cover with aluminium foil and bake in the oven for 40 minutes or until soft.
4. Meanwhile heat a large skillet with the olive oil and fry skin down for 6 minutes on medium high heat. The fat from the skin will render and there will be some excess, tilt the pan and scoop it out with a spoon so the pan stays relatively dry.
5. Turn the breasts over and fry for another 2 minutes. Transfer to the oven and finish cooking the breasts for 3 to 4 minutes.
6. Remove the breast from the pan and allow resting for 5 to 7 minutes.
7. Meanwhile heat the coconut butter in a second pan and heat them through. Turn off the heat.
8. Reheat the duck breast pan, combine the herbs and press the flesh side of the duck breast in the herb mix. Fry for 1 minute, add the maple syrup and reduce into a glaze.lice the duck breast thinly and serve on a bed of veggie and sweet potato, drizzle the maple syrup over the dish to finish.

Nutritional values are manually calculated and based on the ingredients specified.
Nutritional value per serving: Calories: 605.7. Fat: 42.7g Saturated Fat: 10.7g Sodium: 10.1mg Carbohydrate 32.5g Protein: 25.8g Dietary fibre: 2.0g

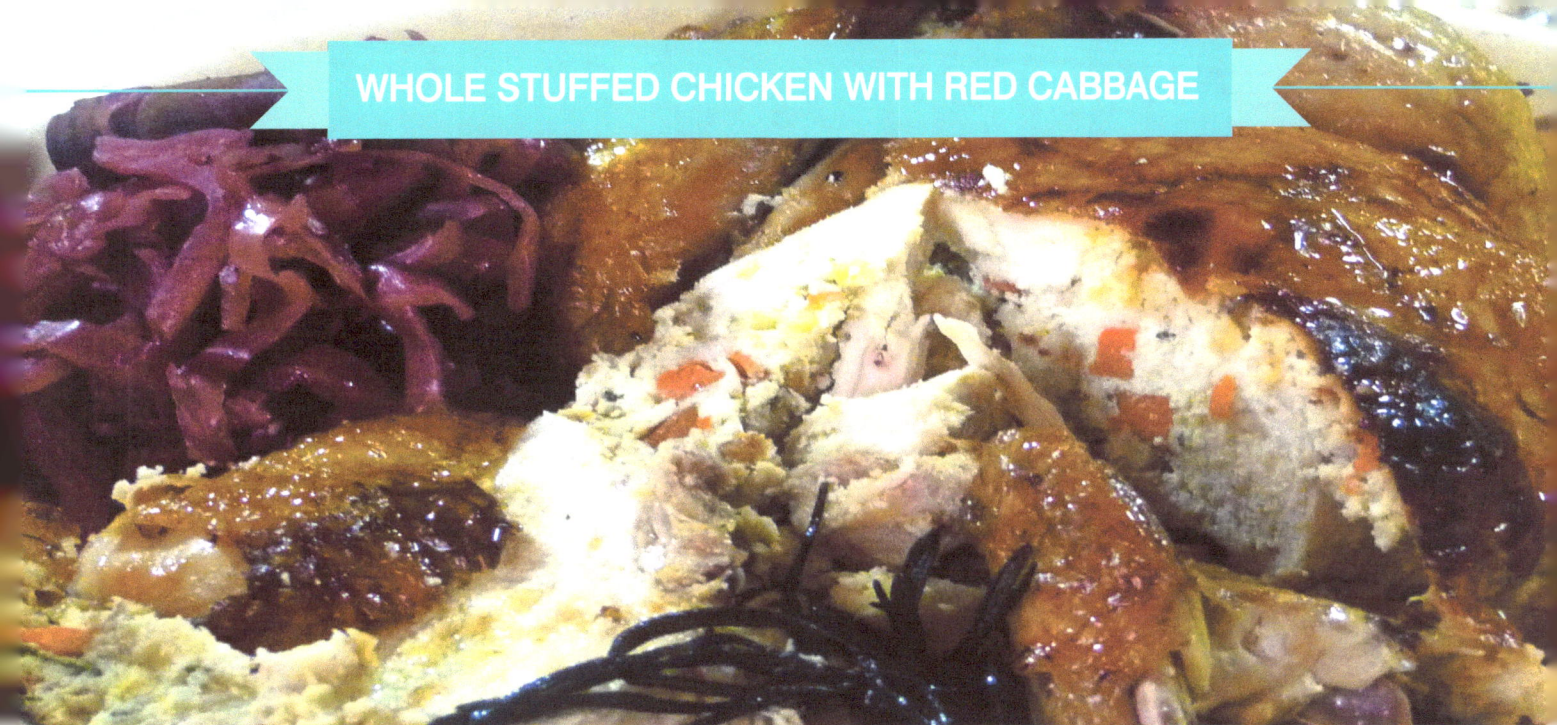

Preparation time: 25 mins

Cooking time: 1 hr 15 mins

Total time: 1 hr 40 mins

This is a nice dish to surprise some friends on a special occasion, or a great meal for a family Sunday lunch! It is a good idea to make friends with your butcher for the preparation, because you need to remove the breastbone from the chicken, without cutting the skin. This is quite easy when you know how, but may be a little tricky until you can master this skill.

Ingredients:

Serves 4

FOR THE CHICKEN:

- 1 whole chicken (1.3 kg, 3 pounds)
- 100gr (3 oz) carrot (cut in small cubes)
- 1 medium onion (finely sliced) • 1 sprig rosemary
- 60ml (2 tbsp) olive oil • 250gr (8 oz) chicken leg meat

- 1 stalk of celery (cut small) • 2 cloves garlic (chopped)
- 30gr (2 tbsp) chopped parsley • Pink salt

FOR THE RED CABBAGE: • Pink salt

- 500gr (2 cups) red cabbage (sliced) • 60 ml (2 tbsp) apple cider vinegar
- 4 cloves • Pink salt • 30gr (1 tbsp) coconut sugar

Method:

1. Cut the chicken leg meat small and place in a food processor, blend fine, add the other ingredients, (except for the chicken and the oil) and pulse to combine.
2. Assuming that your butcher removed the chest bone of the chicken, fill the cavity with the stuffing and press the chicken back into shape.
3. Tie the legs together with a piece of butcher string and place the chicken on a baking tray.
4. Heat an oven to 200 degrees (350 F) and bake the chicken for about 1 hr 15 min. Sprinkle some oil over the chicken after ten minutes for a crispy skin.
5. To be sure that the core is cooked, insert a thermometer if it reaches 73 degrees (170 F) the chicken is cooked.
6. Meanwhile place the cabbage with the other ingredients in a pot, submerge with water and cook until softened, 15 to 20 minutes.
7. Place the chicken on a large serving tray and serve with the red cabbage.

Nutritional values are manually calculated and based on the ingredients specified.
Nutritional value per serving: Calories: 1268.8 Fat: 51.6g Saturated Fat: 10.7g Sodium: 759.4mg. Sugar: 14.1 g
Carbohydrate 31.9g Protein: 163.3g Dietary fibre: 66g

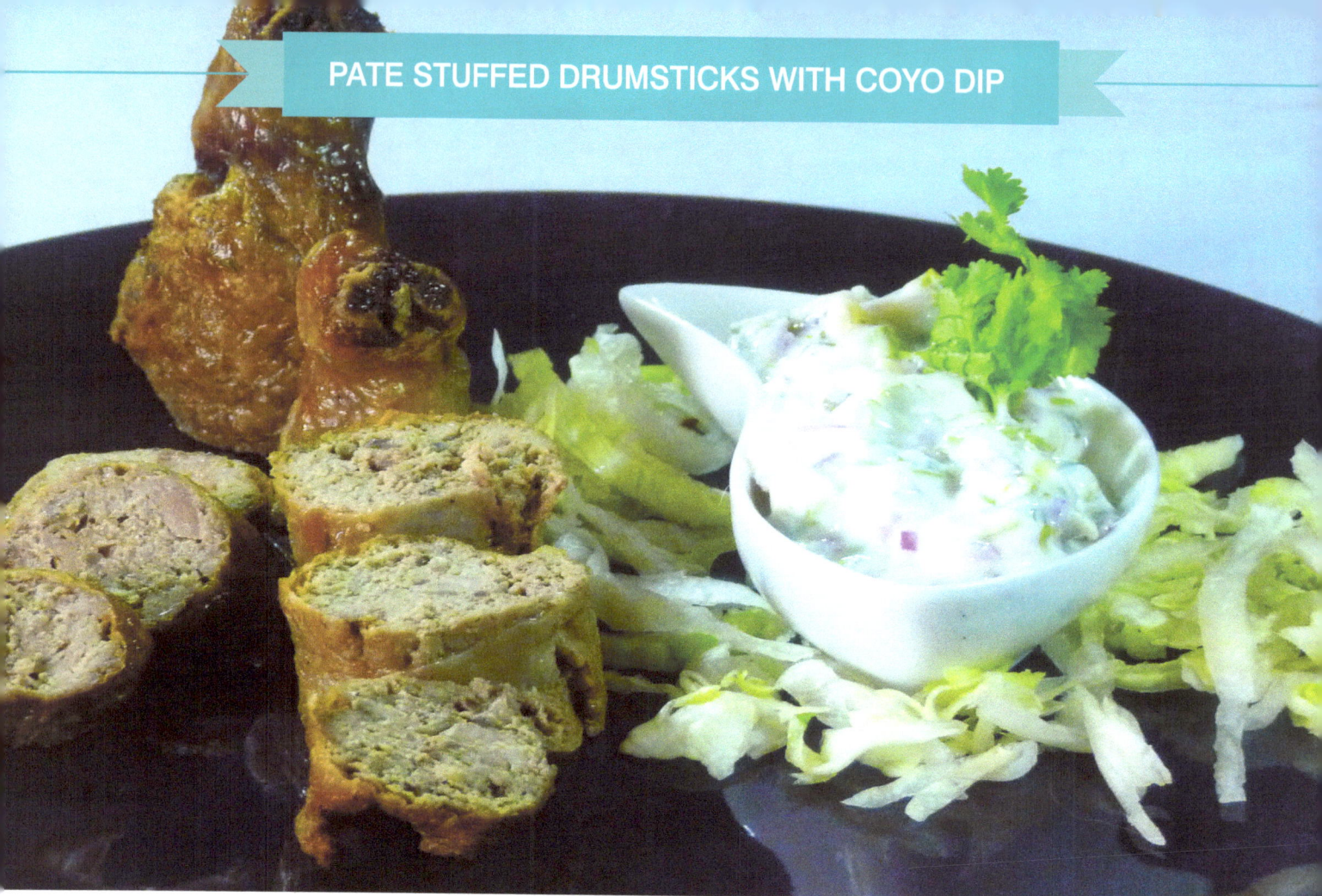

Preparation time: 20 mins

Cooking time: 25 mins

Total time: 45 mins

Snack, lunch or meal? It depends on how you look at it! With the extra nutrition and flavour kick from the livers...bottom line = delicious!

The dish requires a little bit of preparation, but it is luckily not too difficult.

Ingredients: Serves 4

FOR THE DRUMSTICKS:

- 12 drumsticks
- 175gr (6 oz) drumstick meat (cut small)
- 1 medium sized onion (cut small)
- 125 ml (½ cup) coconut cream

FOR THE DIP:

- 60gr (2 tbsp) finely chopped shallots
- 30gr (2 tbsp) cilantro leaves (chopped)

- 350gr (12 oz) chicken liver • Pink salt
- 1 small leek (sliced small)
- 2 cloves garlic (chopped)
- 60 ml (2 tbsp) olive oil

- 12 ml (½ cup) coyo (coconut yoghurt)
- Pink salt

82

(1) Pull with your hands the skin of the drumsticks towards the knuckle.

(2) Once pulled over the knuckle, chop the bone just under the knuckle.

(3) Pull the skin back from the knuckle and put aside.

(4) Remove the meat from the bones and cut small.

(5) Place the meat with the other ingredients, except for the oil, in a food processor and blend together.

(6) Transfer this mix into a piping bag (if you don't have one, use a teaspoon) and fill the skin pockets with the pate.

(7) Fold the edges of the skin around the stuffing and secure with a tooth pick.

(8) Heat the oil in a skillet to low/medium heat, add the drumsticks and fry them golden. They will blow up a bit and maybe the skin will burst, so don't fry too hot.

(9) Transfer the drumsticks to an oven tray and finish baking in a pre-heated oven at 180 degrees (325 F) for 20 minutes. Remove from the oven and allow cooling for a few minutes.

(10) Meanwhile combine the dip ingredients and season with salt.

(11) Serve the drumsticks with the dip and some salad leaves.

Nutritional values are manually calculated and based on the ingredients specified.
Nutritional value per serving: Calories: 436.7. Fat: 23.4g. Saturated Fat: 4.5g. Sodium: 206.4 mg. Sugar: 0.8g Carbohydrate 5.8g. Protein: 48.5.g. Dietary fibre: 0.7 g.

MEAT

BACON ROLLED PORK TENDERLOINS WITH MUSHROOM SAUCE

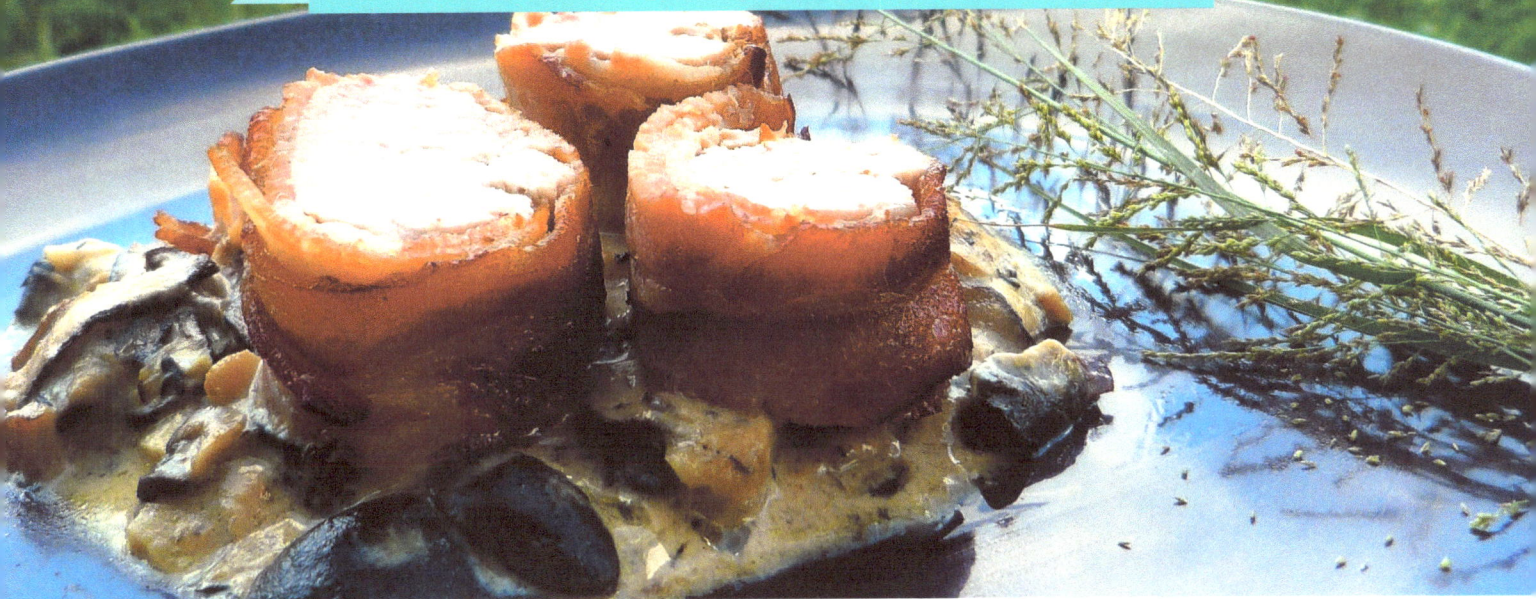

Preparation time: 25 mins

Cooking time: 10 mins

Total time: 35 mins

Just because dairy is no longer in the fridge doesn't mean you have to go without a creamy sauce!
Crispy bacon surrounds tender pork fillet in this recipe, with a good serving of mushrooms and a creamy sauce.

Ingredients: Serves 4

FOR THE PORK:

- 600g (1 ½ pound) pork fillet • 60ml (2 tbsp) olive oil
- 8 rashes smoked bacon • 250ml (1 cup) coconut milk
- Sea salt • 2 sprigs of fresh thyme
- 60ml (2 tbsp) olive oil • 60g (2 tbsp) chopped onions

FOR THE SAUCE:

- 600g (1 ½ pound) mixed mushrooms (cut in bite size pieces)
- 2 garlic cloves (chopped)
- Tapioca flour / water • Pink salt
- 20g (1 tbsp) mushroom powder (If you cannot find it, break dried mushrooms in pieces and grind them in a coffee grinder)

Method:

1. Pre-heat an oven to 180 degrees (325 F)
2. Season the pork fillet with salt and sprinkle the thyme over it.
3. Place the bacon rashes side by side on a flat surface, place the fillet on top and roll the fillet in the bacon.
4. Heat the oil in a skillet to medium heat and fry the fillets for 4 to 5 minutes. Transfer to the oven and finish baking for 10 to 12 minutes. Allow resting for 5 minutes after baking.
5. Meanwhile heat the mushroom oil, in another skillet, to medium heat. Fry the onion and garlic for 2 minutes. Add the mushrooms and fry until cooked and crispy.
6. Remove from the pan and keep aside.
7. Add the coconut milk to the pan, lower the heat and bring to a slow boil, add the mushroom powder and cook for 1 minute, season with a bit of salt and thicken (if needed) with a bit of tapioca flour mixed with water.
8. Slice the pork in 1 ½ cm (¾ inch) slices, arrange the fried mushrooms on plates, top with the pork fillet and drizzle sauce around the plate.

Nutritional values are manually calculated and based on the ingredients specified.
Nutritional value per serving: Calories: 450.3. Fat: 26.7g Saturated Fat: 6.3g Sodium: 1257.3mg. Sugar: 5.6g
Carbohydrate 14.5g Protein: 40.1g Dietary fibre: 1.9g

BEEF ROULADE WITH APPLE SALAD

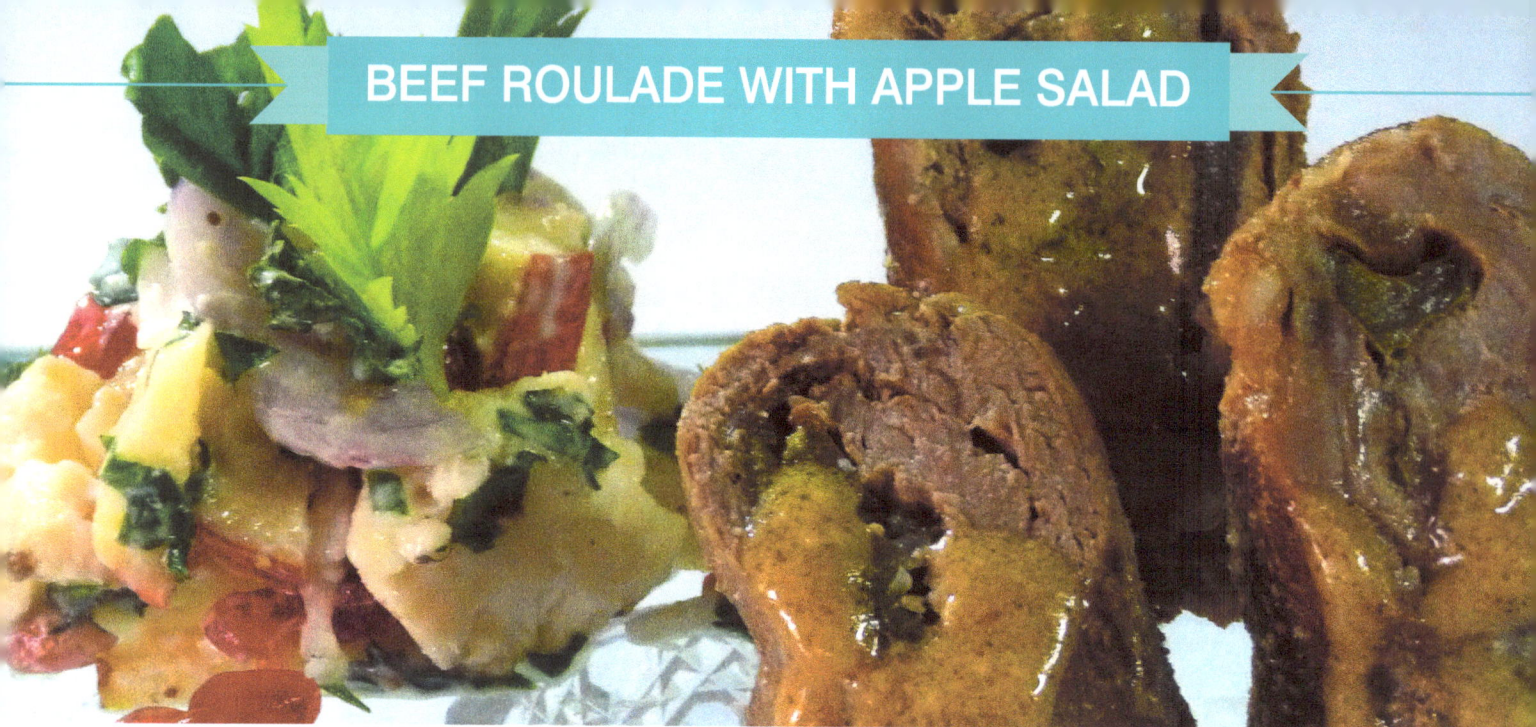

Preparation time: 25 mins

Cooking time: 30 mins

Total time: 55 mins (including chilling time)

This is a dish that looks very impressive but is really simple to prepare! The wide variety of flavours beautifully comes together when the dish is cooked.

Ingredients:

Serves 4

FOR THE PORK:

- 800gr (1 ¾ pound) beef (strip loin, flank steak work well)
- 1 sprig of thyme • 90gr (3 tbsp) shallots (finely sliced
- 60 ml (2 tbsp) olive oil • Pink salt • 1 sprig sage
- 125gr (½ cup) pickled gherkins (cut into small dices) • Bone broth
- 1 sprig rosemary • 125 ml (½ cup) coconut cream

FOR THE SALAD:

- 600gr (2 ¼ cup) apple (cored, quartered and sliced)
- 60gr (2 tbsp) pomegranate • 60gr (2 tbsp) finely chopped shallots
- 125 ml (½ cup) coyo (coconut yoghurt) • Pink salt
- 250gr (1 cup) cauliflower (cut in small florets)
- 30gr (2 tbsp) cilantro leaves (chopped)

Method:

1. Combine the gherkins with the shallots.
2. Ask you butcher to slice the beef in thin slices, so that you get 8 slices.
3. Pound the slices with a tenderizing hammer, place some of the gherkin mix on the broadest end and roll the slices up. Secure the end with a tooth pick.
4. Heat the oil in a skillet to medium high, add the rolls and brown them all around.
5. Add enough bone broth that the rolls are half submerged, add the coconut cream, herbs and cover the pan. Simmer for 20 minutes on low heat.
6. Meanwhile prepare the salad by combining all ingredients in a bowl, season if needed, and chill.
7. Remove the beef roulade from the pan, strain the gravy and reduce to desired thickness.
8. Remove the tooth picks from the beef roulades and arrange them on plates, drizzle with the gravy and serve with the chilled salad.

Nutritional values are manually calculated and based on the ingredients specified.
Nutritional value per serving: Calories: 668.1. Fat: 40.7g Saturated Fat: 14.5g. Sodium: 341.1 mg. Sugar: 17.3g. Carbohydrate 29.1 g. Protein: 48.3.g. Dietary fibre: 2.7 g.

BRAISED PORK WITH CELERIAC LASAGNE, SPINACH AND BONE BROTH GRAVY

Preparation time: 10 mins	Cooking time: 45 mins	Total time: 55 mins

Lasagne - that's not AIP! With a little imagination you can create amazing dishes on AIP.
Tender cooked pork is layered with spinach and slices of celeriac. An easy to make dish, healthy, tasty and it looks amazing.

Ingredients: Serves 4

FOR THE PORK:

- 1750g (1 ½ pound) pork meat, (shoulder or blade is great for this dish)
- 3 cloves garlic (crushed)
- 1 stalk of celery (roughly cut)
- 250 ml (1 cup) bone broth
- 1 sprig rosemary
- 60 ml (2 tbsp) olive oil
- 1 small carrot (cut in slices)
- 1 medium onion (cut in quarters)
- Pink salt

FOR THE SPINACH:

- 1 kg (2 ½ pound) raw spinach
- Pink salt
- 2 cloves garlic (grated)

FOR THE GRAVY:

- Pink salt
- 500 ml (2 cups) bone broth

FOR THE LASAGNE:

- 12 thin slices celeriac
- 1 medium onion (finely sliced)
- 60 ml (2 tbsp) olive oil

Method:

1. Heat the oil for the pork in a Dutch oven. Season the pork with salt, add to the pan and brown on both sides until well caramelized. Add the vegetables and rosemary and fry for another minute. Add the broth, bring to a boil, lower the heat, cover the pot and braise until the pork is fork tender. (40 minutes or so).
2. Bring the bone broth to a boil in a saucepan, lower the heat and reduce on low heat until about 125 ml (½ cup). Meanwhile boil the celeriac slices in water with a little salt until soft, 3 to 4 minutes. Drain, rinse and keep aside.
3. Remove the spinach leaves from the stems and set aside. Heat the oil in a skillet, add the onion and garlic and fry for 1 minute.
4. Add the spinach leaves and fry until wilted and softened, season and keep warm.
5. When the pork is fork tender, pull it apart so you get small strands of meat.
6. Place a slice of celeriac on a plate, top with spinach, followed by pulled pork meat, repeat with another layer. Top with another slice of celeriac and drizzle gravy around the plate.

Nutritional values are manually calculated and based on the ingredients specified.
Nutritional value per serving: Calories: 857.6. Fat: 62.1g Saturated Fat: 16. 8g Sodium: 437.9 mg. Sugar: 1.8g
Carbohydrate 30.8g Protein: 48.4g Dietary fibre: 7.9g

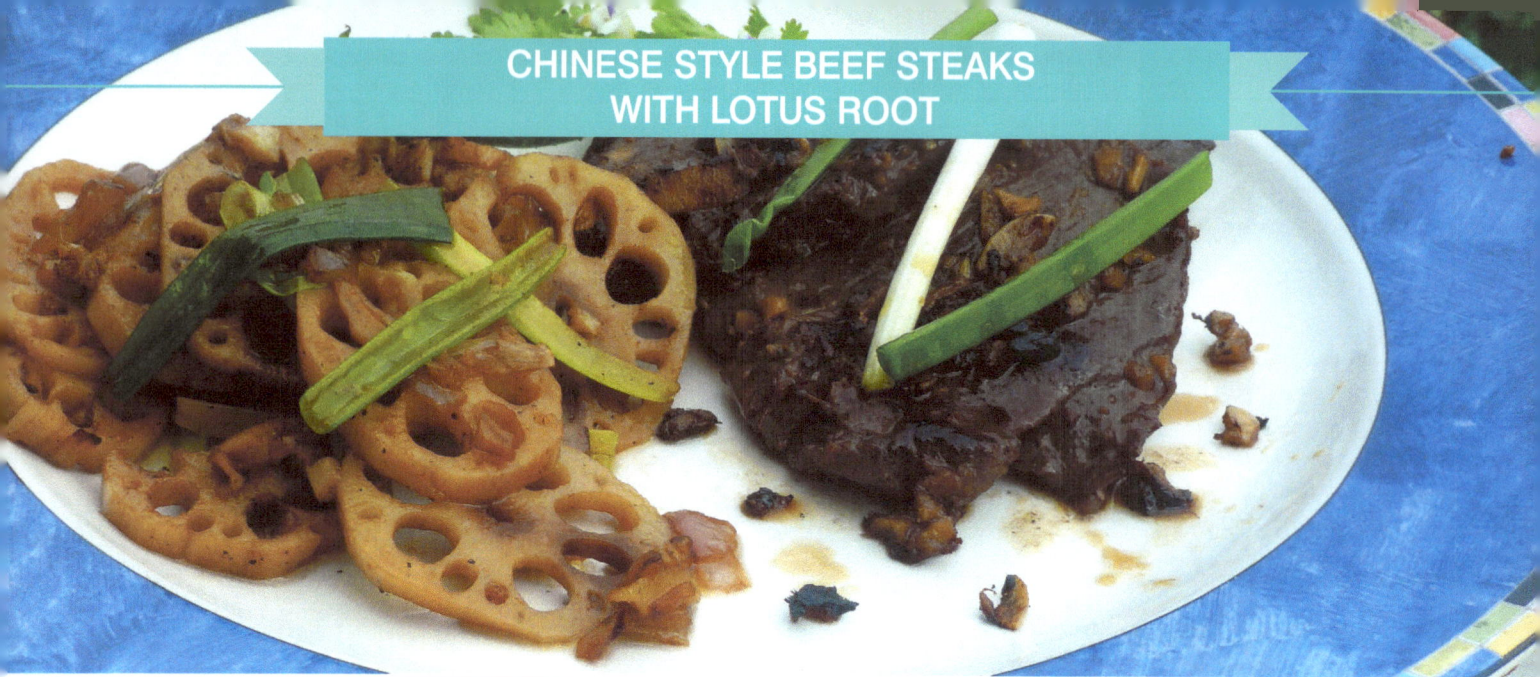

Preparation time: 25 mins

Cooking time: 10 mins

Marinating Time: 1 hr

Total time: 1 hr 35 mins

Lotus root may not be a vegetable you are used to seeing or eating, however this root vegetable has many health benefits. It is high in fibre, vitamin C and B group vitamins. It has a great crunchy texture with a slightly sweet taste and takes on flavours well. A fantastic vegetable to help mix things up a bit on AIP! You will find lotus root readily at Asian food stores or local markets. Sometimes if the fresh root isn't available you can also get it frozen.

Ingredients: Serves 4

FOR THE STEAKS:

• 600g (1 ½ pound tender beef) sliced in 12 small steaks

• 60g (2 tbsp) coconut aminos • 90ml (3 tbsp) olive oil

• 60g (2 tbsp) grated young ginger

• Pink salt • 90ml (3 tbsp) olive oil

• 3 cloves garlic (chopped)

FOR THE LOTUS ROOT:

• 450g (1 pound lotus root)

• 60ml (2 tbsp) coconut aminos • Vinegar for the lotus root

• 3 stalks spring onion (cut in 5 cm, 2 inch, long pieces)

• 30g (1 tbsp) chopped garlic

• 60 ml (2 tbsp) olive oil • 30g (1 tbsp) grated young ginger

Method:

1. Place the steaks with the ginger, garlic and aminos in a bowl and mix, add a little salt if needed. Allow marinating for one hour.
2. Lotus root turns almost immediately brown after you peel the skin, so prepare a bowl of water with some vinegar to prevent this.
3. Peel the lotus root with a vegetable peeler and slice thinly, about ½ cm (¼ inch) thick and add to the vinegar water.
4. Heat the olive oil for the steaks in a skillet on high heat, add the steaks and fry them quickly, 1 minute on each side.
5. Heat the oil for the lotus root in another skillet on high heat, add the garlic and ginger and stir for a few seconds. Add the lotus root slices and fry for a few minutes. The lotus root will become translucent when cooked.
6. Add the spring onions. Season with the aminos.
7. Place three steaks on plates and serve the lotus root on the side.

Nutritional values are manually calculated and based on the ingredients specified.
Nutritional value per serving: Calories: 536.4. Fat: 41.3g Saturated Fat: 13.0g Sodium: 414.8mg. Sugar: 0.1g Carbohydrate 21.8g Protein: 31.4g Dietary fibre: 2.4g

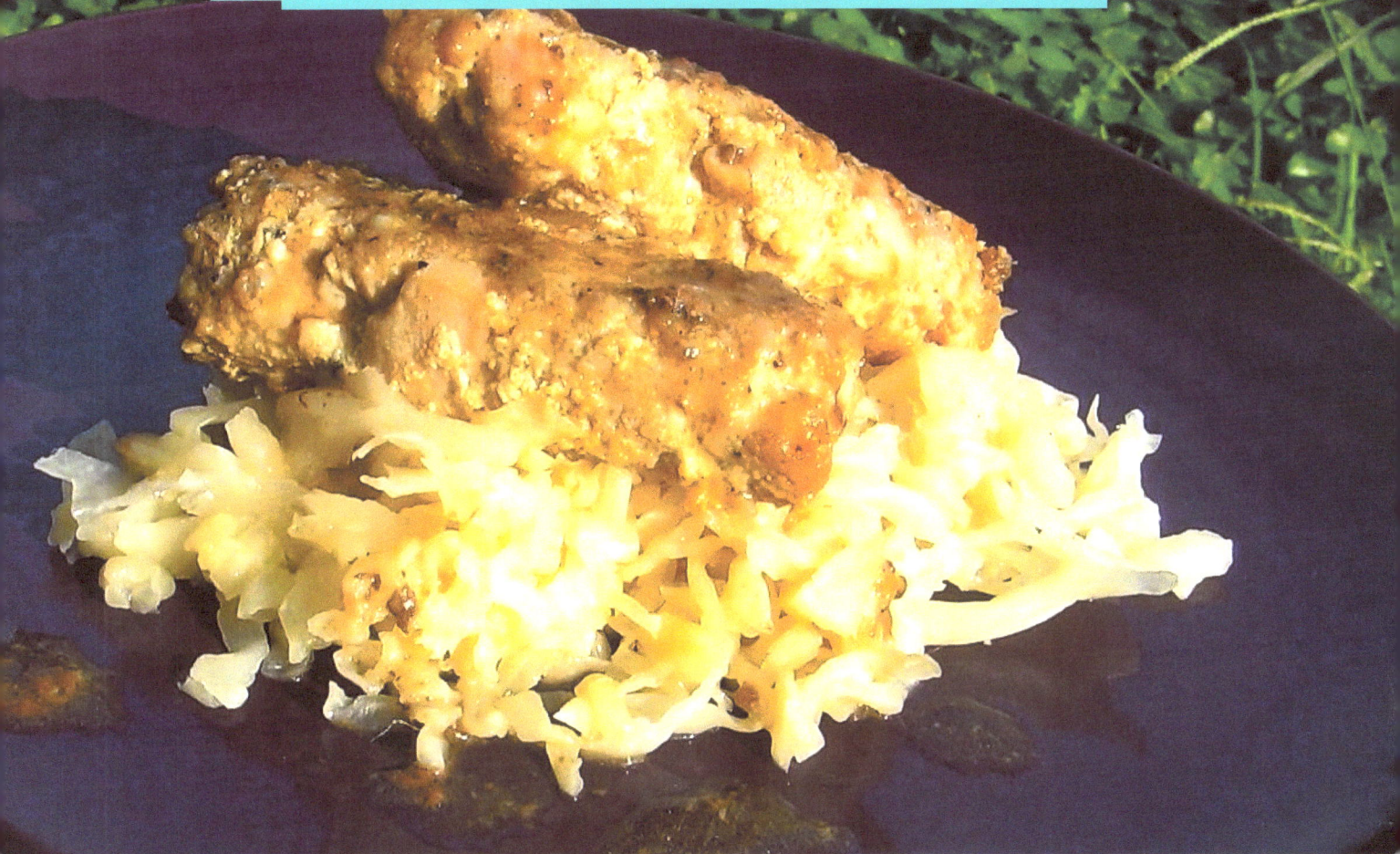

Preparation time: 20 mins

Cooking time: 15 mins

Total time: 35 mins

I have European heritage and nothing feels like comfort food to me like sauerkraut and bangers. It evokes memories of my Dad making food from "back home". These are some of my most beloved food memories. Fermented foods are nutrient dense super foods to include in your diet, packed full of gut healing goodness. This is a perfect recipe for batch cooking. You can make a larger batch of bangers and freeze them. Sauerkraut can be made in large batches and keeps well in the fridge.

Ingredients: Serves 4

FOR THE SAUERKRAUT:

- 1kg (2 ½ pounds) sauerkraut

- 4 cloves

FOR THE BANGERS:

- 600g (1 ½ pound) 30% fat minced pork

- 200 g (6 ½ oz) pork liver (coarsely chopped)

FOR THE SAUSAGE SPICE MIX:

- 15g (1 tsp) dry parsley flakes

- 30g (2 tsp) onion powder   • 7g (½ tsp) pink salt

- 15g (1 tsp) dry thyme   • 15g (1 tsp) garlic powder

- 30 g (1tbsp) spice mix   • 60ml (2 tbsp) lard

- Pork net fat (ask your butcher)

Method:

1 Combine all dried spices and store the balance in a container and keep in a dry place for later use.

2 Ensure the minced pork and liver are very cold, place in a mixing bowl, add the spice mix and combine.

3 It is best to knead the sausage mix with your hands, after 2 to 3 minutes you will feel that the mix firms up; this is due to activation of the protein.

4 If you want to check the mix for taste, just make a small ball and fry or boil. Let the mix cool in the fridge for ½ hour.

5 Add just enough water to cover the sauerkraut. Add the cloves and boil for 15 to 20 minutes.

6 Pork net fat is the membrane that surrounds the stomach of pigs. It is a great tool to hold your sausages in shape when frying. Ask your butcher they will have some, or can get you some. It freezes well so you can keep the leftovers for later use.

7 Spread a piece of the neck out on a flat surface. Divide the sausage mix into 8 equal portions.

8 Shape the mix like a sausage about 10 cm (2 ½ inch) long and place on the net. Roll the net around the meat ensuring it is nicely shaped, then cut away excess net. The net will practically disappear when the sausages are fried so if there is a bit extra around the meat, no harm done.

9 Heat the lard in a skillet, add the sausages and fry them on medium heat for 4 to 5 minutes on both sides.

10 Drain excess water from the sauerkraut and divide over plates, top each plate with 2 bangers and drizzle with some of the lard from the skillet.

Nutritional values are manually calculated and based on the ingredients specified.
Nutritional value per serving: Calories: 536.4. Fat: 41.3g Saturated Fat: 13.0g Sodium: 414.8mg. Sugar: 0.1g Carbohydrate 21.8g Protein: 31.4g Dietary fibre: 2.4g

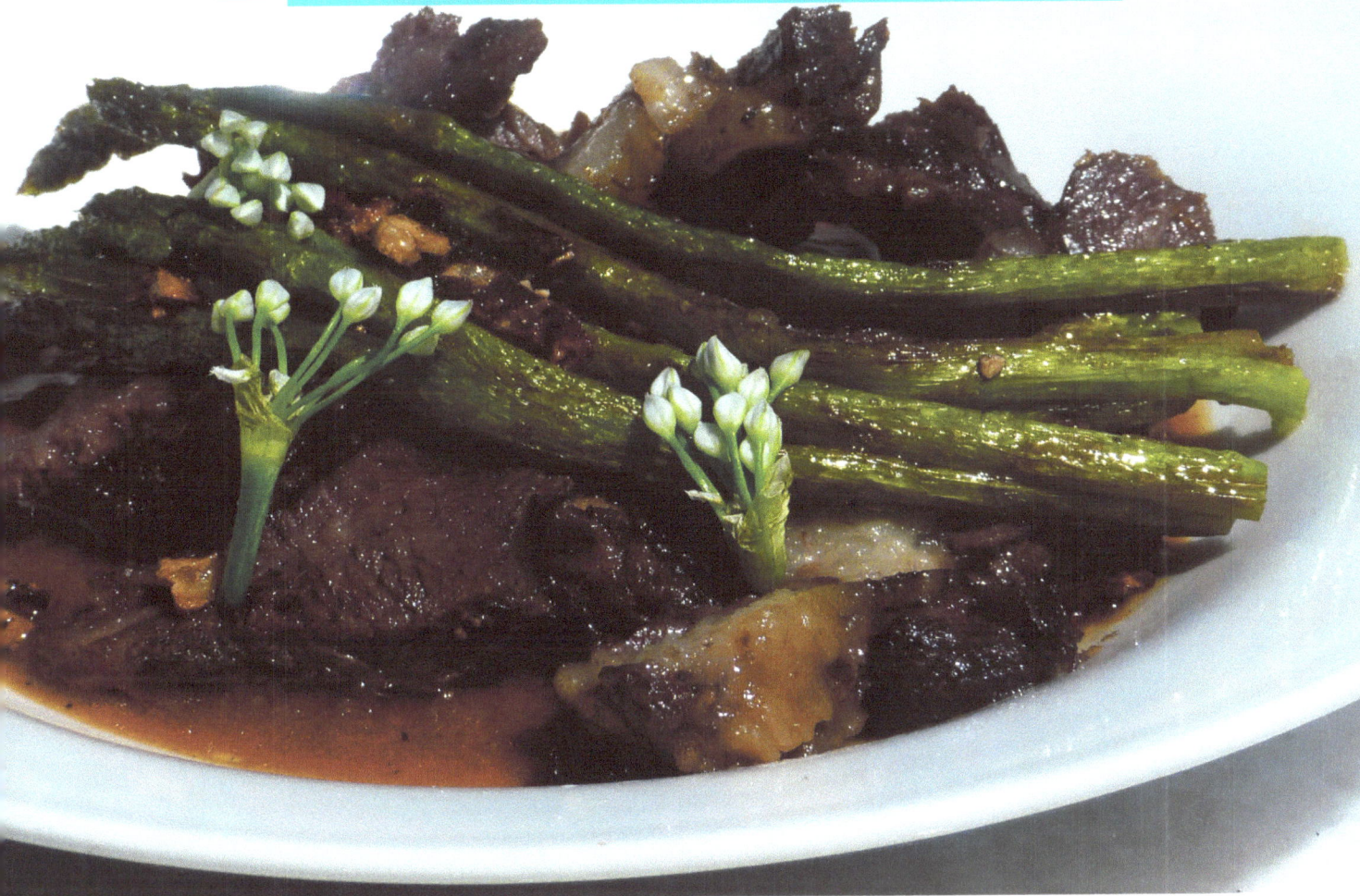

Preparation time:
15 mins

Cooking time:
1 hr 30 mins

Total time:
1 hr 45 mins

Slow braising the tougher cuts of meat can not only taste awesome; but is very economical as well. As a bonus you get all the extra goodness from the connective tissues. For this recipe I have combined the intense flavours of the stew with a delicate vegetable. The asparagus can handle the intensity of the stew very well. Feel free to experiment by adding some of your favourite root veggies too!

This also makes for a great batch cooking dish that will freeze well. When reheating serve with your favourite greens.

Ingredients:

Serves 4

- 900gr (2 pounds) lamb shoulder

- 4-5cloves garlic (sliced)

- Small bunch of thyme

- Pink salt   • 2 sprigs rosemary

- 375 ml (1 ½ cup) bone broth

- 450gr (1 pound) fine green asparagus

- 1 medium onion (roughly cut)

- 90 ml (3 tbsp) olive oil

Method:

1. Heat 2 table spoons of the oil in a Dutch oven on medium heat, add the onion, garlic and fry for 1 minute.

2. Add the meat, some salt and the rosemary and thyme.

3. Fry the meat until browned.

4. Add the bone broth, cover the pot and simmer on low heat until the meat is fork tender.

5. When the meat is done, remove from the pan and strain through a sieve.

6. If needed, reduce the sauce until it sticks to a spoon.

7. Meanwhile heat a griddle to high heat.

8. Clean the asparagus by snapping off the base about 5 cm (2 inches) from the bottom.

9. Combine the asparagus with the remaining oil, a little salt and the 2 cloves of garlic.

10. Grill the asparagus 3 to 4 minutes on the griddle.

11. Portion the lamb shoulder and divide over plates, top with asparagus and drizzle the sauce over the dish.

**Nutritional values are manually calculated and based on the ingredients specified.
Nutritional value per serving:** Calories: 602.5. Fat: 37.6g Saturated Fat: 11.7g Sodium: 268.3mg. Sugar: 0.4g Carbohydrate 13.7 g Protein: 51.7g Dietary fibre: 3.1g

MARINATED LAMB CHOPS WITH STIR FRIED PAK CHOY AND BABY CARROTS

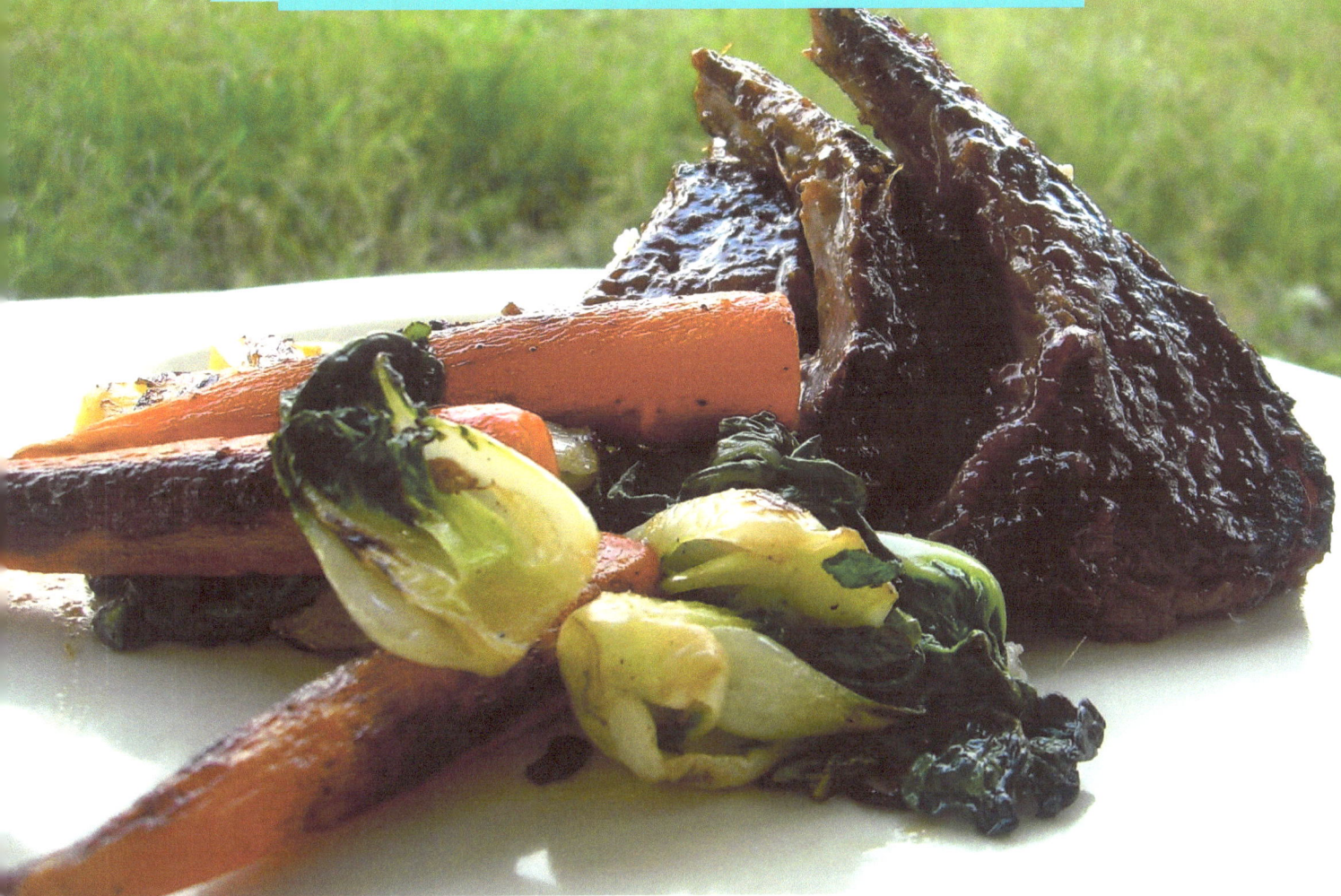

Preparation time: 15 mins

Cooking time: 15 mins

Marinating Time: 2 hr

Total time: 2 hr 30 mins

This is a summer BBQ dish! Succulent juicy lamb chops and grilled veggies are the perfect match for a BBQ meal!

Ingredients: Serves 4

FOR THE LAMB:

- 12 Lamp Chops 70g (2 1/2 oz) each

FOR THE MARINADE:

- Juice from 1 lime
- 2 sprigs rosemary

FOR THE VEGGIES:

- 300g (0.6lb or 10.5oz) baby carrots
- 2 cloves garlic (chopped)
- Pink Salt

- 3 cm fresh ginger (grated)
- 70ml (2 ½ oz) coconut aminos
- 2 cloves garlic (minced)
- Arrowroot

- 500g (1.1lb) pak choy
- 1 medium onion (chopped)
- 2 tbsp olive oil

Method:

1. Combine the marinade ingredients, without the arrowroot.

2. Marinate the lamb chops in half of the marinade for at least 2 hours.

3. Remove the lamb chops from the marinade.

4. Add the other half of the marinade and bring to a soft boil and simmer for 5 minutes. Mix a bit of arrowroot with some water and thicken the marinade into a glaze. Remove from the heat.

5. Remove the bases of the pak choy and cut into 1 cm pieces. Peel the baby carrots.

6. Grill the carrots on a greased pre-heated grill until soft, 3 to 4 minutes.

7. Heat the olive oil in a skillet on medium heat and add the onion and garlic and fry for 1 minute.

8. Add the chopped pak choy and stir fry for 1 minute. Season. Lower the heat and simmer for 2 minutes (if necessary add a bit of water to avoid drying up or burning).

9. Grill the lamb chops on a greased pre-heated grill, applying the glaze with a brush during the cooking process.

10. Apply some more glaze after the lamb chops are cooked for a shiny presentation.

11. Arrange the veggies on a serving tray and top with the lamb chops.

Nutritional values are manually calculated and based on the ingredients specified.
Nutritional value per serving: Calories: 548.6. Fat: 29.7g Saturated Fat: 11.4g Sodium: 1193.1mg Carbohydrate 22.9g Protein: 45.1g Dietary fibre: 2.9g

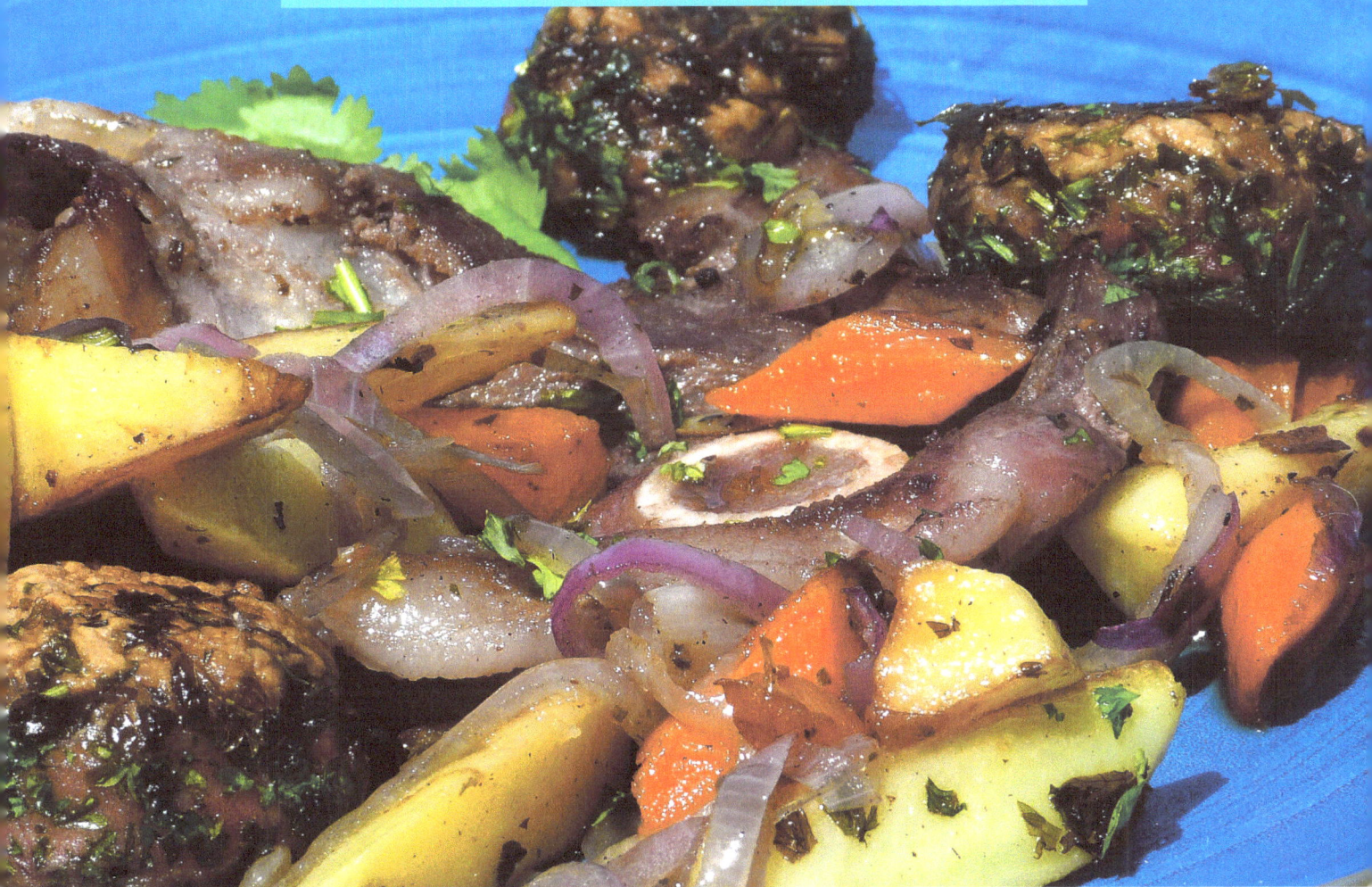

Preparation time: 25 mins

Cooking time: 20 mins

Total time: 45 mins

A pretty, tasty and exiting meal! This dish is a nutritional powerhouse! There is a bit of preparation involved, but once you are all set the finished dish comes together quite quickly.

Ingredients: Serves 4

FOR THE LAMB:

- 650g (1 ½ pound) lamb chops, use loin chops or shoulder chops

FOR THE VEGETABLES:

- 2 medium sized sweet potatoes (peeled and cut into wedges)
- 300g (0.6lb or 10.5oz) baby carrots
- 60ml (2 tbsp) olive oil
- FOR THE LIVER BALLS:

- 15g (1 tsp) dried rosemary
- Pink salt   • 30ml (1 tbsp) olive oil

- 450g (1 pound) baby carrots (cut into small pieces)
- 1 large red onion (cut into half- moon rings)
- 1 medium onion (chopped)

- 120g (4 oz) liver of your choice (beef, pork, chicken, lamb)
- 60ml (2 tbsp) olive oil
- 90g (3 tbsp) chopped parsley
- 120g tapioca starch

FOR THE GRAVY:

- 450ml bone broth
- 30ml (1 tbsp) coconut aminos

Method:

1. Cook the sweet potatoes and carrots separately in water with a little salt for 5 minutes or until softened but still firm. Drain, rinse cold and keep aside.

2. Cut the liver in small pieces, place in an up-right blender and blend smooth with a little salt.

3. Transfer to a bowl, add the tapioca starch and combine into a dough like consistency; the starch added looks like a lot, but will be quickly absorbed.

4. Season the lamb chops with salt, rosemary and the olive oil.

5. Place the bone broth with the aminos in a small sauce pan and reduce until about ½ a cup on low heat.

6. Form small balls from the liver (wet hands help make this a lot easier). Coat the liver balls with the parsley and fry them for 5 minutes on medium heat in a skillet with the oil.

7. Fry the sweet potatoes golden brown for about 5 minutes in the oil, add the carrot and onions half way through this process.

8. Lastly fry the lamb chops for 2 minutes on both sides, allow to rest for 2 to 3 minutes.

9. To assemble arrange the potato/veggie mix on the plates and place the lamb chops in the centre. Arrange the liver balls around the chops and drizzle some of the reduced gravy over the dish.

Nutritional values are manually calculated and based on the ingredients specified.
Nutritional value per serving: Calories: 809.3. Fat: 59.5g Saturated Fat: 14.8g Sodium: 161.2mg. Sugar: 1.5g Carbohydrate 35.3g Protein: 49.8g Dietary fibre: 3.6g

PORK FILLET WITH MUSHROOMS AND SWEET POTATOES

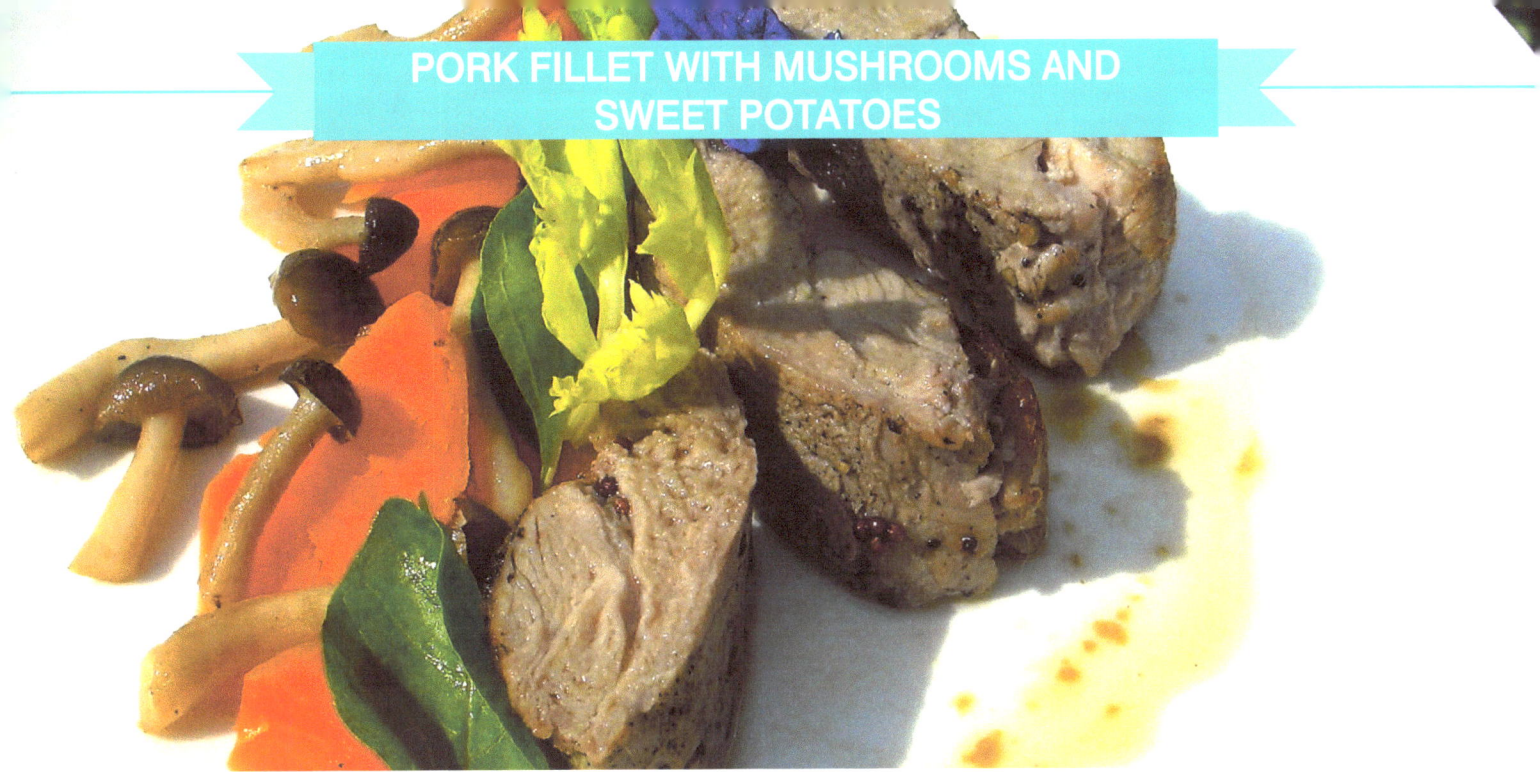

Preparation time: 10 mins

Cooking time: 15 mins

Total time: 25 mins

Tender juicy pork loin is a real treat and cooks very quickly. A dish that is easy but does not skimp on flavour! Paired with lovely tasting mini cremini (baby Portobello) mushrooms and sweet potatoes this recipe makes a dish to savour.

Ingredients:

Serves 4

- 750g (1 ½ lbs) pork tenderloin
- 600g (2 ¼) cups sweet potatoes • Pink salt
- 500g (2 cups) Buna Shimoji mushrooms
- 250ml (1 cup) bone stock • 60g (2 tbsp) olive oil

Method:

1. Pre-heat an oven to 180 Celsius (325 F).
2. Peel and wash the sweet potato and cut into wedges.
3. Boil the sweet potato wedges in water with a little salt until they soften, about 5 minutes. Drain and keep aside.
4. At the same time, place the bone stock in a small sauce pan, bring to a boil, lower the heat and simmer until reduced to ¼ cup.
5. Heat the olive oil in a skillet to medium high heat, add the fillet and fry until browned all around. About 2 minutes. Transfer the fillets to a baking tray and finish baking in the oven for 10 minutes. Transfer the fillets to a plate and allow to rest under aluminium foil for 5 minutes.
6. Re-heat the skillet, add the mushrooms and fry until cooked, about 30 seconds. Remove from the pan and keep aside.
7. Add the drained sweet potatoes to the pan and fry for 2 minutes.
8. Slice the pork fillet crosswise in 1 inch thick slices and place them on individual plates. Arrange the mushrooms and sweet potato around it and drizzle some gravy over the meat.

Nutritional values are manually calculated and based on the ingredients specified.
Nutritional value per serving (12 slices per cake): Calories: 485.3 Fat: 12.4g Saturated Fat: 3.0g Sodium: 106.7mg Carbohydrate 30.6g Protein: 73.1g Dietary fibre: 2.1g

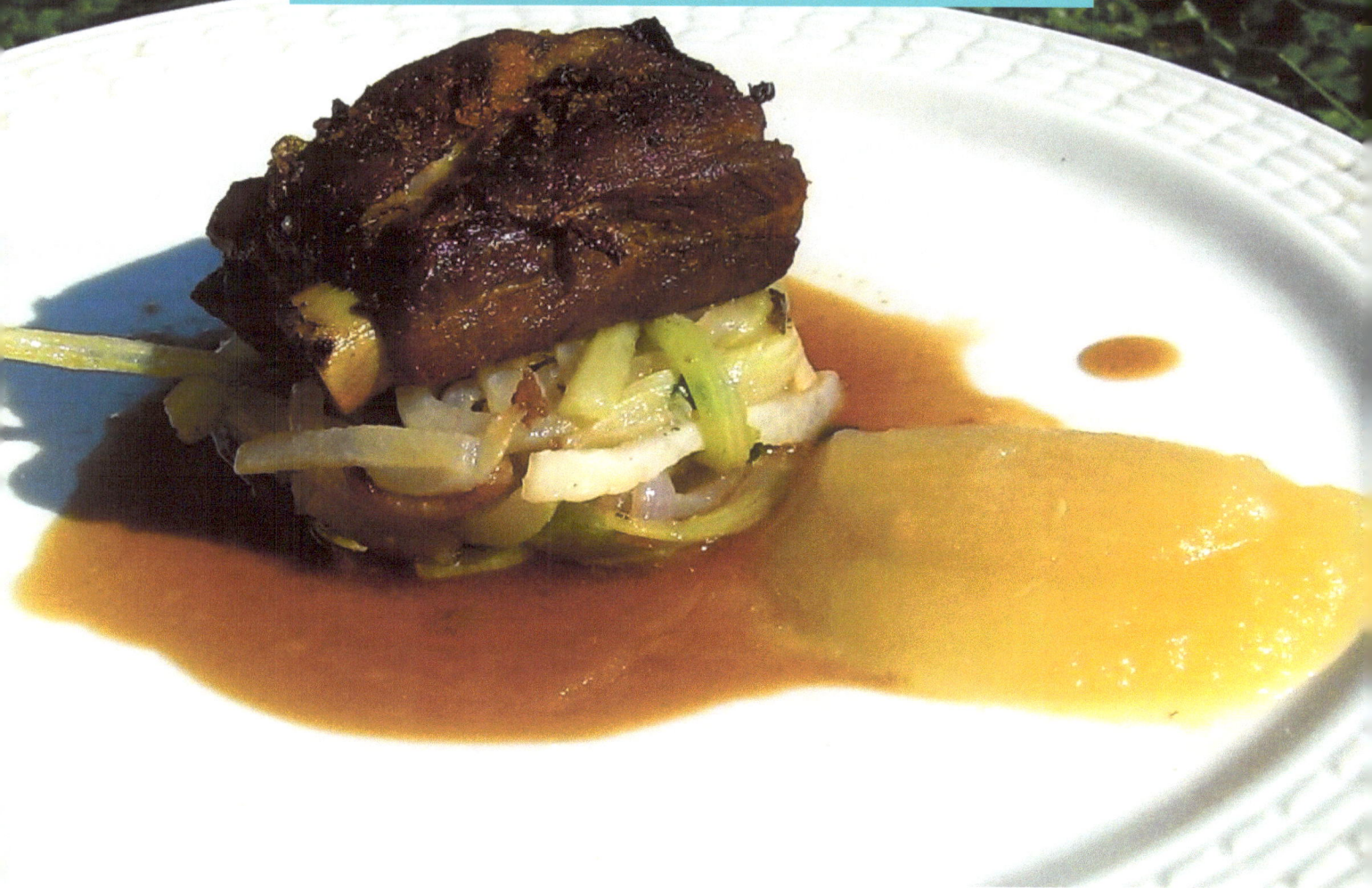

Preparation time:
1 hr

Cooking time:
2.5 hrs

Total time:
3.5 hrs

We know how challenging it can be when you are on AIP, thinking about what you are going to eat when visiting friends or going on outings. In Australia, BBQ's with family and friends are very much a part of our lifestyle, especially in summer. This can make AIP a bit more challenging, however this gorgeous dish will ensure your friends ask you for the recipe, and is perfect for a Summer BBQ. It just smells and looks so good.

Make a larger batch of these short ribs and store them in the freezer after cooking along with the delicious stock. These pork short ribs are perfect to then take to a BBQ with your family or friends, simply ensure they are defrosted before heating them. This two way style of cooking in this recipe is an advantage.
This recipe needs a little preparation but the finish is quick and easy.

Ingredients: Serves 4

FOR THE SHORT RIBS:

* 1kg (2 ½ pound short ribs

* 1 stalk of celery (roughly cut)

* ½ medium size onion

* 1 medium size carrot (roughly chopped)

- 250ml (1 cup) home- made chicken broth
- Sea salt
- 2 bay leaves
- 30gr (1 tbsp) ground turmeric

- 60ml (2 tbsp) lard
- Palm oil for deep frying

FOR THE VEGETABLES:

- 2 stalks celery (cut in 8 cm, 3 ½ inch long strips)
- 60g (2 tbsp) olive oil
- 150g (5oz) radish (cut in 8 cm, 3 ½ inch long strips)
- 1 medium red onion (sliced into half moons)
- 30g (2 tbsp) fresh cilantro leaves, or parsley

FOR THE APPLE PUREE:

- 1 large apple
- Juice of ½ a lime

Method:

1. Divide the short ribs into 4 equal portions.

2. Day 1 - Heat the lard in a Dutch oven on medium heat. Season the ribs with a little salt and fry them until browned on all sides. Add the carrot, celery, chicken stock and bay leaves, braise on low heat until the ribs are cooked, about 1 to 1 ½ hours. You should be able to easily pierce a knife through.

3. Remove the ribs from the pan, allow cooling and store in the fridge.

4. Strain the stock through a fine sieve or cheese cloth and place this also in the fridge. Discard the veggies.

5. Boil the apple with a little water and the lime juice until soft, about 5 minutes. Blend smooth and store in the fridge as well.

6. Day 2 - Slice the vegetables in strips.

7. Heat a deep fryer to 180 degrees (325 F).

8. Scoop the fat, which has now hardened on top of the stock; preserve the fat for later use. You will now have a jelly like stock.

9. Combine the ground turmeric with a little water to create a paste. Brush the paste all over the ribs. If you have made a larger batch of ribs store the remainder at this point for later use.

10. Heat the olive oil in a skillet to medium heat in a skillet and fry the vegetables until softened, 3 to 4 minutes. Season to taste.

11. Deep fry the ribs until golden brown, about 3 minutes, drain on kitchen paper.

12. Scoop some jelly stock on plates followed by the vegetables. Top with the fried ribs and a spoonful of apple puree on the side.

Nutritional values are manually calculated and based on the Ingredients specified.
Nutritional value per serving: Calories: 989.3 Fat: 74.9g Saturated Fat: 27.7g Sodium: 88.1mg
Carbohydrate 11.9g Protein: 63.5g Dietary fibre: 3.0g

ROAST PORK WITH SPROUTED BROCCOLI

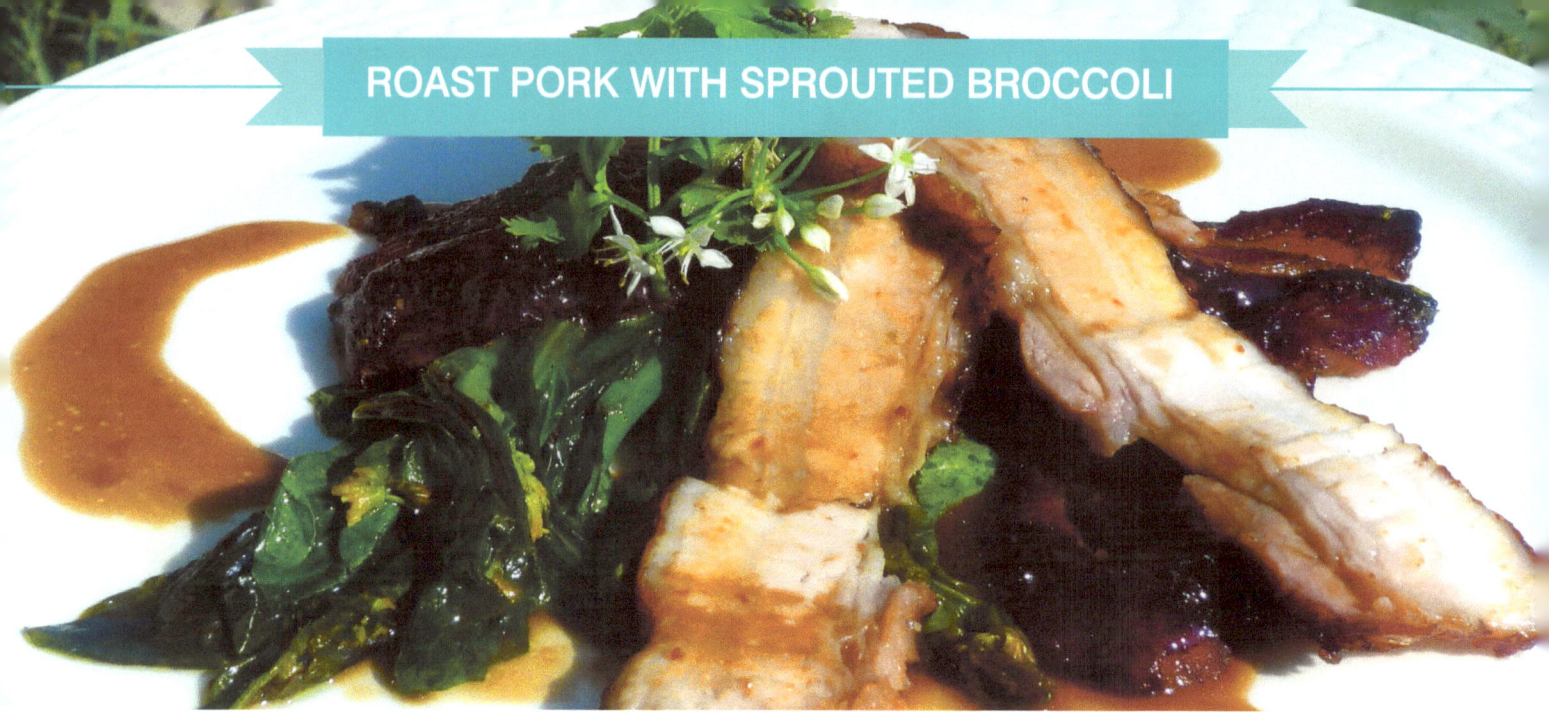

Preparation time: 10 mins	Cooking time: 45-60 mins	Total time: 1 hr

This is a great dish for pork lovers! Shoulder or belly work equally as well, however, I love pork belly. I love the flavour of Coconut aminos; it totally kicks soy sauce to the curb! The aminos give the pork a beautiful colour and flavour once roasted. If you are using a belly cut ensure that you don't marinade the skin if you want crackling! Just liberally sprinkle the rind with pink salt and give it a final blast at 200 degrees for approx 20 mins, once the meat is nice and fork tender. The vegetables combine well with the pork and the marinade which functions as a sauce.

Ingredients: Serves 4

- 800g (2 pounds) pork (shoulder or belly works well)
- 750g (1½ pound) sprouted broccoli
- 60ml (2 tbsp) olive oil
- 2 cloves garlic (grated)
- 1 medium onion (finely sliced) • Pink salt
- 200g (7 oz) coconut amino

Method:

1. Place the pork with the coconut amino, half of the onion, and garlic in a bowl and marinade for 2 hours.
2. Place the pork on an oven tray and roast in a pre-heated 200 degree (375 F) oven for 45 minutes, or until fork tender. Reserve the leftover marinade.
3. Heat the oil in a skillet to medium heat add the onion and garlic, fry for 30 seconds, add the broccoli and fry for another 2 minutes.
4. Add a little water and cook until the vegetables have softened on low heat, 5 to 7 minutes. Meanwhile bring the marinade to a boil in a sauce pan, lower the heat and reduce until it looks like a thin glaze.
5. Arrange some broccoli stalks on plates, top with sliced roasted pork and drizzle with the sauce.

Nutritional values are manually calculated and based on the ingredients specified.
Nutritional value per serving: Calories: 737.9 Fat: 45.5g Saturated Fat: 15.9g Sodium: 809.9mg Sugar: 0.0g Carbohydrate 17.6g Protein: 62.8g Dietary fibre: 6.0g

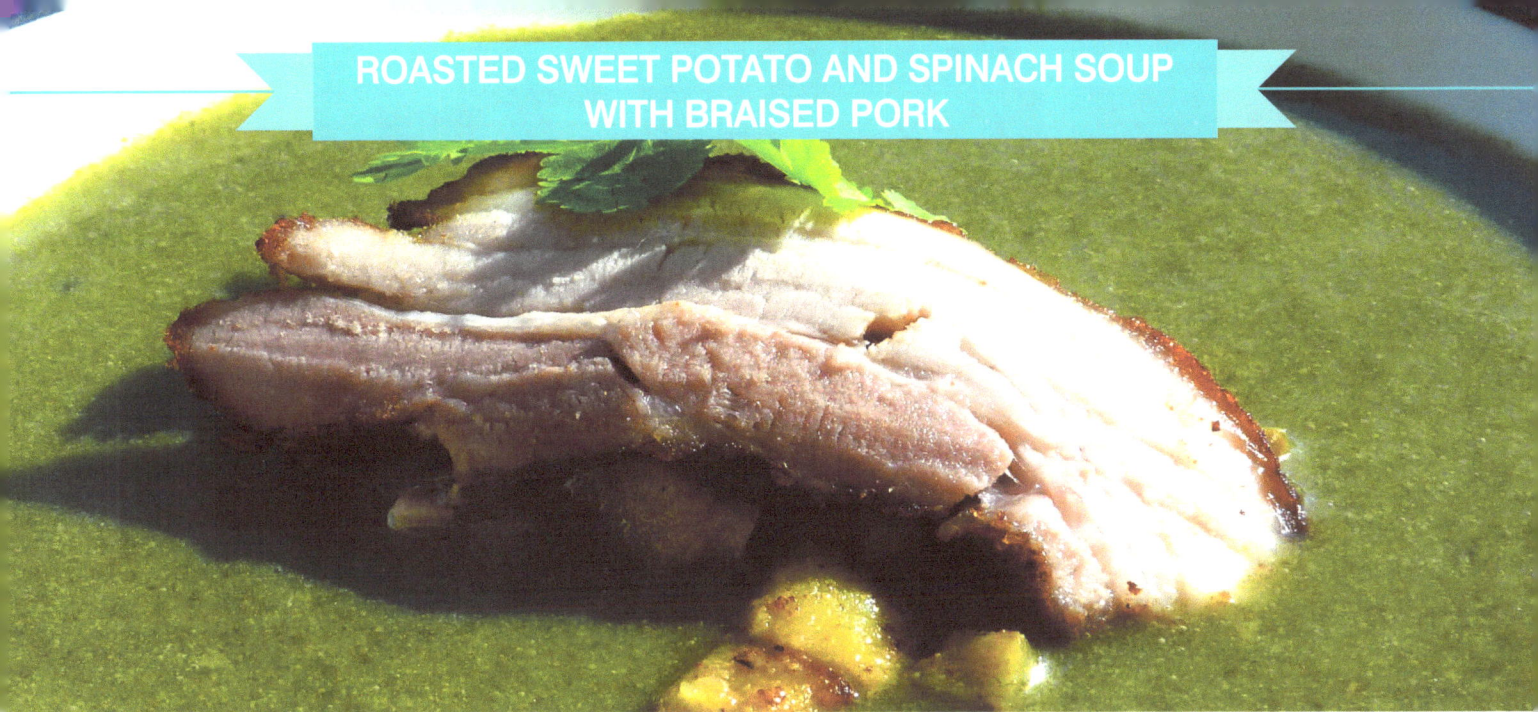

ROASTED SWEET POTATO AND SPINACH SOUP WITH BRAISED PORK

Preparation time: 20 mins

Cooking time: 30 mins

Total time: 50 mins

A delicious hearty soup full of nutrients and the braised pork gives the soup a nice twist. You can make a larger batch of the soup, portion pack and freeze. Just add slices of cooked bacon to the soup and freeze together.

Ingredients: Serves 4

- 450g (1 pound) sweet potato (cut into cubes)
- 1 medium onion (roughly cut)
- 250g (8 oz) pork belly rind removed
- 1ltr (4 cups) bone broth

- 750g (1 ½ pound) spinach leaves and stems
- 2 cloves garlic • 90ml (3 tbsp) olive oil
- 250 ml (1 cup) bone broth • Sea salt
- 30g (1/4 cup) chopped cilantro leaves

Method:

1. Place the pork belly with the one cup of bone broth in a small sauce pan, cover and braise for 30 or so minutes on low heat. When the pork can easily be pierced through with a knife it is cooked. Leave to cool in the stock, allow to cool completely in the fridge for easy slicing later.
2. Place the sweet potato with the onion and garlic on an oven tray, sprinkle with the oil and roast in a pre-heated 200 degree (375 F) oven for 12 to 15 minutes.
3. Place the spinach in a large pot; add the roast mix, plus the bone broth and the leftover bone broth from the pork. Bring to a boil, lower the heat and cook for 15 minutes.
4. Transfer the mix to an up-right blender and blend smooth. Secure the lid of the blender by holding it in place with a kitchen towel.
5. Return the soup to the pot, season and serve hot with a slice of the braised pork belly.

Nutritional values are manually calculated and based on the ingredients specified.
Nutritional value per serving: Calories: 786.9. Fat: 47.0g Saturated Fat: 16.5g Sodium: 481.3 mg Sugar: 2.6g Carbohydrate 55.6g Protein: 40.5g Dietary fibre: 8.3g

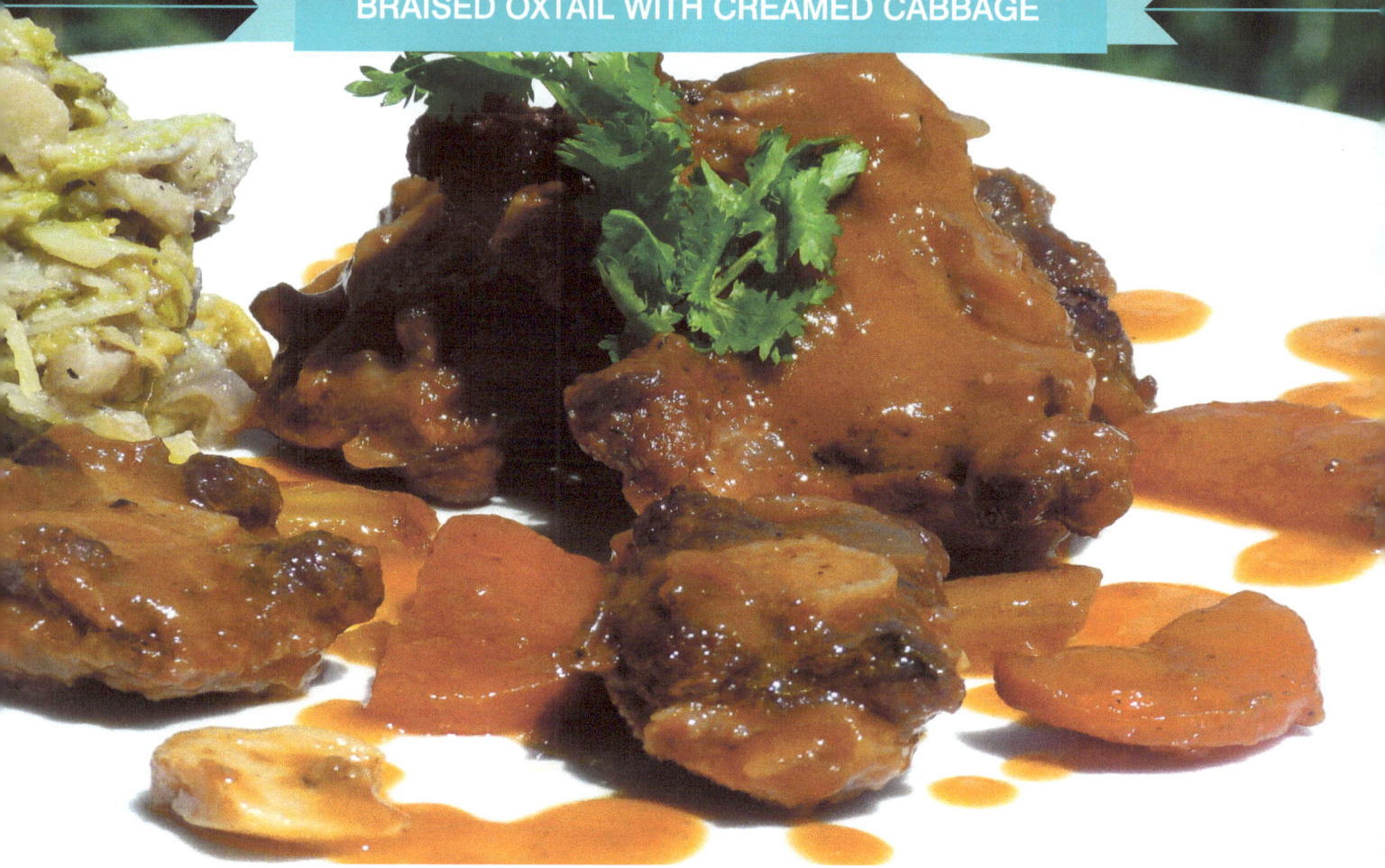

Preparation time: 15 mins	Cooking time: 1 hr 30 mins	Total time: 1 hr 45 mins

Thick, rich tomato heavy ox tail ragu was one of my favourite meals before going AIP. I would fight my brother in law for the bones, sucking up all the succulent marrow! Braising meat is very time consuming so this makes for a perfect slow cooker meal, and you can easily make a big batch to freeze.

The cuts suitable for braising are full of muscle and collagen, adding so much flavour and goodness to dishes.

Ingredients: Serves 4

- 2 large red onions (roughly cut)
- 1.5 kg (3 ½ pounds) oxtail (cut into slices)
- 1 large carrot (sliced)   • Sea salt
- 3 cloves garlic (chopped)   • 90 ml (3 tbsp) olive oil

- 30gr (1 tbsp) dried thyme
- 1 large of stalk celery (cut in 2 cm, 1 inch) pieces
- Small bunch of parsley roughly chopped
- 250 ml (1 cup) bone broth

FOR THE CABBAGE:

- 900gr (2 pounds) sliced cabbage
- 1 medium onion (finely sliced)

- Pink salt
- 250 ml (1 cup) coconut cream
- 90 ml (3 tbsp) olive oil

Method:

1. Pre-heat an oven to 180 degrees (325 F).

2. Season the oxtail with salt and the thyme.

3. Heat the oil in a large skillet and fry the oxtail until browned on both sides,

4. Add all the vegetables and fry for 1 minute.

5. Transfer the meat/vegetable mix in a braising pan or slow cooker. Add the bone broth, cover the pan and braise in the oven for 1 and ½ hrs; or until the meat is fork tender. If needed add some more bone broth.

6. Meanwhile heat the oil for the vegetables in a stockpot. Add the onions and fry for 30 seconds, then add the cabbage and fry for another 2 minutes until the cabbage starts to wilt. Add the coconut cream, lower the heat, cover the pan and simmer for 10 minutes.

7. When the oxtail is fork tender remove the meat from the pan and keep aside. Remove the vegetables with a slotted spoon from the liquid in the pan and transfer to an up-right blender. Blend smooth.

8. Return the mix to the pan and strain through a fine sieve.

9. Divide the oxtail over plates, place some vegetables on the side and spoon the gravy over the dish.

10. Serve hot.

Nutritional values are manually calculated and based on the ingredients specified.
Nutritional value per serving: Calories: 1070.3. Fat: 85.7g Saturated Fat: 30.2g Sodium: 352.0mg. Sugar: 3.3g Carbohydrate 27.1g Protein: 53.6g Dietary fibre: 7.4g

BEEF STEW

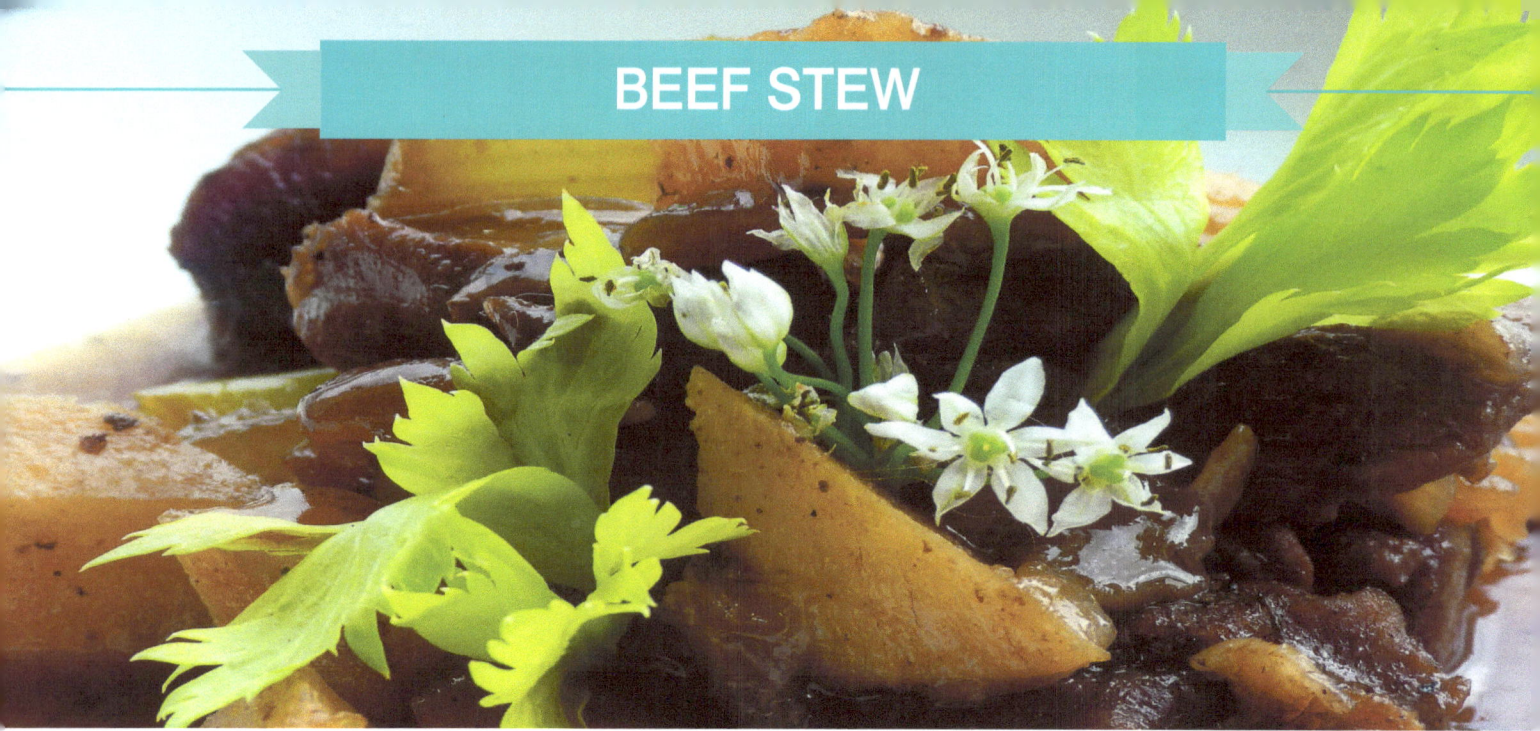

Preparation time: 25 mins

Cooking time: 5 hrs

Total time: 5 hrs 25 mins

If time constraint is an issue, or like me you often struggle with having little energy, it is time to get the slow cooker out of the cupboard! It has saved me so many times! Throw everything in the pot, set on low and when you come back from work it is done. This is also another perfect meal for batch cooking. Amazing smells will greet you as you walk through the door!!

Ingredients: Serves 4

- 600 g (1 ½ pound) stew beef (chuck works fine)
- 150 g (5 oz) sweet potatoes • 150 g (5 oz) carrots
- 1 medium onion • Small bunch of thyme
- 20 g (1 ½ tbsp) chopped parsley
- 60 ml (2 tbsp) olive oil

- Half bulb of garlic skinned and roughly chopped (I love garlic, so use how much you prefer)
- Pink salt • 150 g (5 oz) parsnips
- 150 g (5 oz) pumpkin
- 150 g (5 oz) celery
- 2 bay leaves • 750 ml (3 cups) bone broth

Method:

1. Cut the beef and all the vegetables in to chunky pieces.
2. Heat the oil in a skillet on high heat.
3. Season the beef with salt and the thyme.
4. Add the seasoned beef to the pan and fry until browned. Add the vegetables and fry for another minute, mixing well.
5. Add the broth and bay leaves and bring to a boil.
6. Transfer the mix to a slow cooker and cook until you come home, at least 5 hours.
7. If the liquid is still thin, thicken with a little tapioca starch mixed with some water.
8. Serve hot.

Nutritional values are manually calculated and based on the ingredients specified.
Nutritional value per serving: Calories: 521.7. Fat: 19.4g Saturated Fat: 6.7g Sodium: 343.9mg. Sugar: 4.3g Carbohydrate 39.4g Protein: 47.9g Dietary fibre: 5.3g

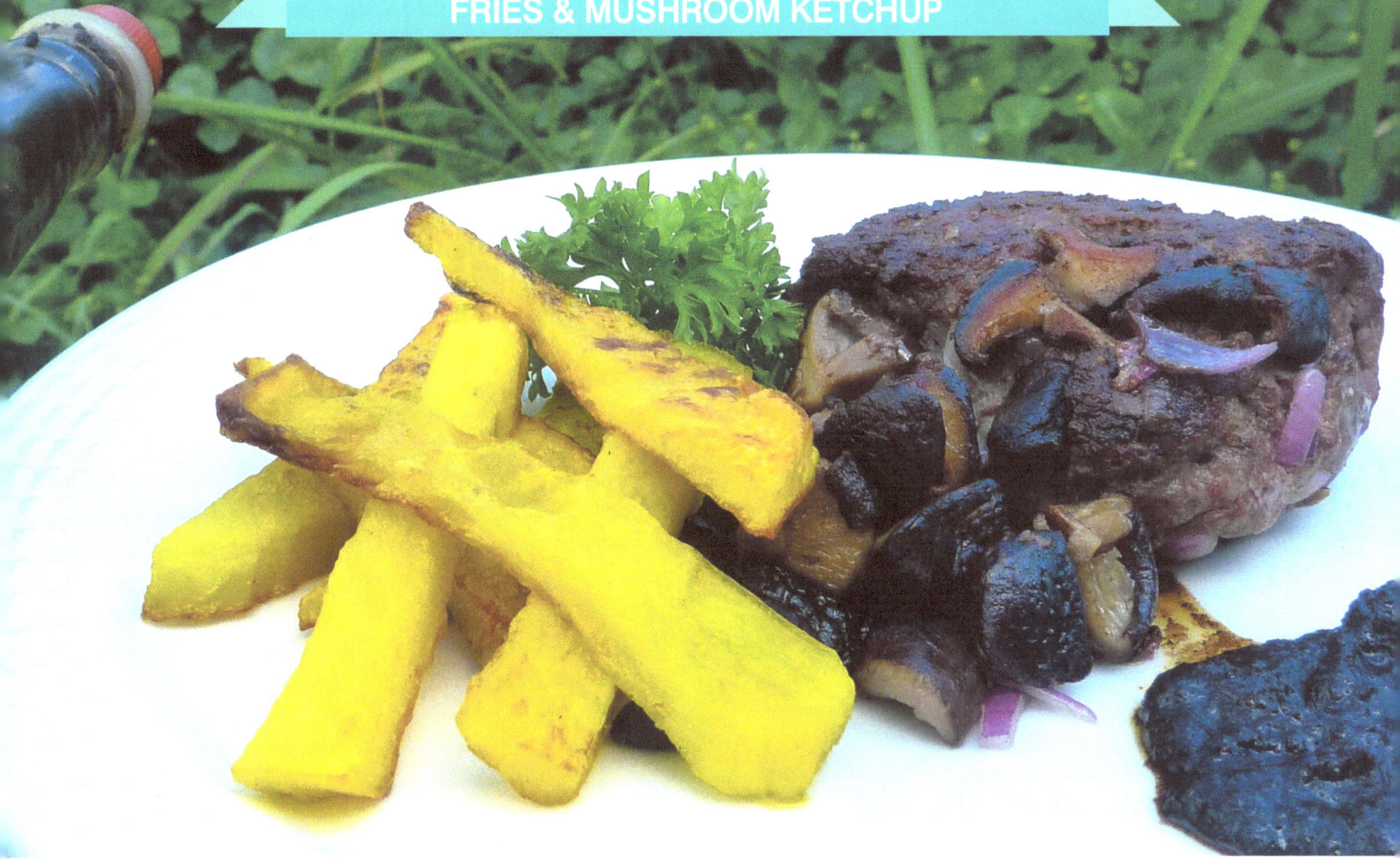

Preparation time: 20 mins	Cooking time: 15 mins	Total time: 35 mins

Who cannot get excited over a good burger? This deconstructed AIP version is sure to bring back those juicy burger memories! Mushroom ketchup!? Yup!! This is a real flavour surprise that pairs well with all meats!! Served with sweet potato fries, this recipe is indeed a feast to savour.

Ingredients: Serves 4

FOR THE BURGERS:

- 600g (1 ¼ lbs) minced beef   • 60g (2 tbsp) olive oil

- 450g (1 pound) sweet potato(cut into fries sticks)

- 2 cloves garlic, finely chopped

FOR THE KETCHUP: 1 BATCH (1.8 LITRE/ 3 PINTS)

- 2.7 kg (6 pounds) button mushrooms

- 1.2ltr (2 pt) vinegar   • 5g (1 tsp) ginger

- 12pcs big size Shi-take mushrooms (chopped)

- 60g (2 tbsp) chopped onion

- 2 tsp turmeric powder   • Pink salt

- 175g (6 oz) salt

- 5g (1 tsp) mace

- 2.5g (½ tsp) cloves

Method:

(1) To make the ketchup: Break the mushrooms into small pieces and sprinkle with the salt, leave for 12 hours or overnight.

(2) Rinse the mushrooms; add the vinegar and spices and simmer in a covered saucepan for 30 minutes or until most of the vinegar has been absorbed.

(3) Blend the mixture in an upright blender and press through a sieve after blending.

(4) Pour the ketchup into warm bottles or containers and sterilize for 30 minutes in boiling water. The ketchup will easily last for a year.

(5) Combine the minced meat with salt, chopped onion, mushrooms and garlic. Mix well and allow resting for 15 minutes in the fridge.

(6) Slice the sweet potatoes lengthwise in ½ cm (1/4 inch) thick slices, make the slices about 10 cm (2 ½ inch) in length and slice them into fries shapes. Sprinkle with the turmeric powder and mix well.

(7) Form 4 patties from the minced beef.

(8) Heat the olive oil on a griddle to high heat and fry the patties 3 to 4 minutes on each side, time depends on how well you like them cooked.

(9) Meanwhile heat an oven to 200 Celsius (375 F).

(10) Fry the fries crisp and golden in 10 to 15 minutes, in the oven on a baking tray, mix them with some salt.

(11) Place a burger on plates, and serve with fries and the ketchup.

Nutritional values are manually calculated and based on the ingredients specified.
Nutritional value per serving (12 slices per pattie): Calories: 601.6 Fat: 36.2g. Saturated Fat: 3.0 g. Sodium: 1084.2mg. Carbohydrate: 16.8g. Protein: 53.4g. Dietary fibre: 4.1g.

SSAMBAP

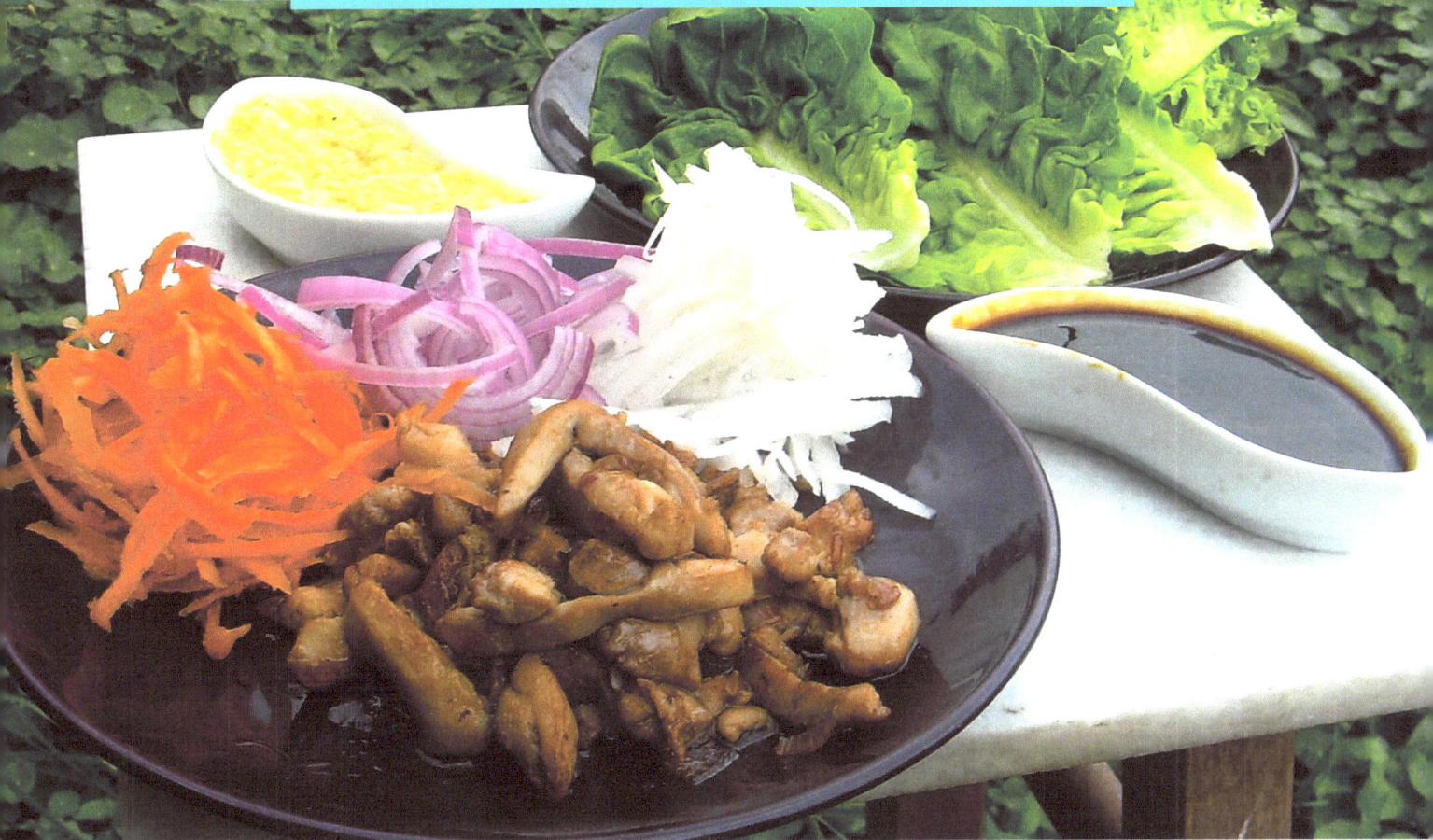

Preparation time: 35 mins

Cooking time: 05 mins

Total time: 40 mins

Here in Australia, Asian cuisine and style of cooking is extremely popular. It is one of my favourite cuisines to cook! Nutritious, fresh, very tasty and easy to prepare. Ssambap literally means 'Wrap' in Korean. Delightfully seasoned grilled meat is cut into small strips and stir fried, then scooped into crunchy salad leaves and topped with a little sauce!! I gave the original a little twist to make it AIP compliant.

Ingredients: Serves 4

FOR THE SSAMBAP: 900gr (2 pounds) pork meat, if you want it tender use fillet, but lean leg meat works fine as well. Cut into strips. Any other meat works also e.g. chicken or beef.

- ½ medium size onion (finely chopped)

- ½ cup coconut aminos
- 250gr (1 cup) shredded carrot
- 3 cloves garlic (grated)

- 60gr (2 tbsp) olive oil
- 250gr (1 cup) shredded radish

Equivalent to 1 head of lettuce or mixed salad leaves (lettuce, red leave lettuce, escarole, romaine) just make sure the leaves are shaped so that they can hold the meat.

FOR THE SAUCES:

- 250ml (1 cup) coconut aminos

- Arrowroot

- 2 cloves garlic (minced)

- SAUCE 2:

- 125gr (½ cup grated ginger) • Pink Salt

- Juice of ½ a lemon

Method:

1. Place the meat strips in a mixing bowl, add the onions, garlic and coconut aminos and mix well. Cover the bowl and marinade for 2 hours or overnight.

2. Meanwhile bring the coconut aminos with the garlic to a soft boil in a sauce pan, thicken with arrowroot mixed with a little water.

3. If you find the coconut amino taste too strong use half water, half aminos. Allow cooling time.

4. For sauce 2: Combine the ginger with the lemon juice and season with a little salt. You should have a 'soggy' ginger pulp.

5. Heat the olive oil in a large skillet to high heat.

6. Remove any excess marinade from the meat and stir fry for 2 to 3 minutes. The best way to stir fry the meat is in a few batches, to avoid the meat being steamed instead of fried.

7. Place all ingredients in separate serving bowls and arrange on the dinner table.

8. Take a salad leave in your hand; add a little carrot, a little radish, then some meat, and lastly some sauce. Fold the salad and … enjoy.

Nutritional values are manually calculated and based on the ingredients specified.
Nutritional value per serving: Calories: 540.6. Fat: 18.8g Saturated Fat: 4.8g Sodium: 11.92mg
Carbohydrate 18.2g Protein: 67.9g Dietary fibre: 3.4g

BBQ CHICKEN AND PORK SKEWERS WITH CUCUMBER SALAD

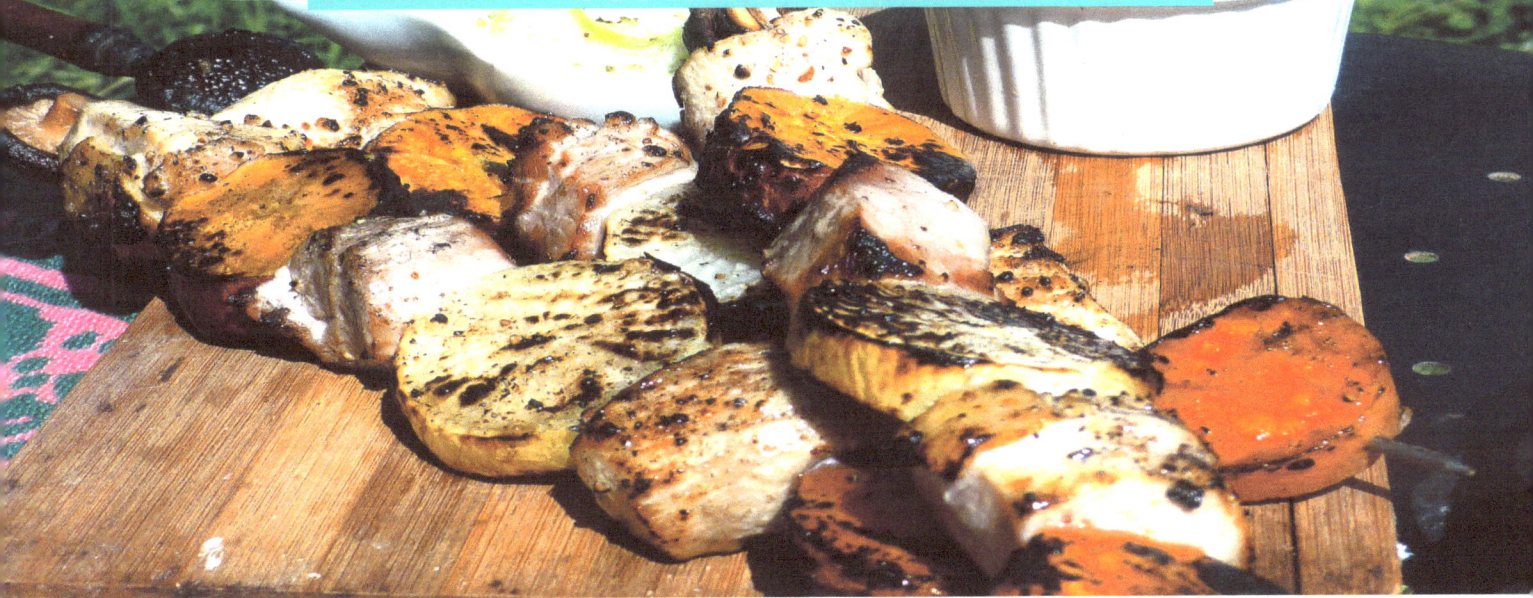

Preparation time: 35 mins	Cooking time: 15 mins	Total time: 50 mins

What is a BBQ without some skewers? All those smoky charred bits, juicy meat and crunchy veggies, yum! This recipe shows that you don't have to be deprived of great BBQ food when following AIP. Great meat lovely vegetables and a refreshing salad, no worries just happy people.

Ingredients: Serves 4

FOR THE SKEWERS:

- 300gr (10 oz) chicken legs skin-on (cut into chunky pieces)
- 100gr (3 oz) radish (cut into 1 cm, ¾ inch, slices)
- 15gr (1 tbsp) rosemary
- 300gr (10 oz) pork meat (cut into chunky pieces)
- Pink salt
- 100gr (3 oz) orange sweet potato (cut into 1 cm, ¾ inch, slices)

- 12 button mushrooms
- 100gr (3 oz) carrots (cut into 1 cm, ¾ inch, slices)

FOR THE SALAD:

- 600gr (1 ½ pound) cucumber (peeled and thinly sliced)
- 60ml (2 tbsp) coconut mayonnaise
- 30gr (1 tbsp) salt
- 15gr (1 tbsp) chopped dill

Method:

1. First place the rosemary into some oil; we will later use this as a brush to grease the skewers.
2. Next is the salad. Slice the cucumber thinly on a mandolin and mix with the salt, allow standing for 15 minutes.
3. Meanwhile boil the hard vegetables, (carrot, sweet potato, and radish) for 3 to 4 minutes in water, to soften them a bit, or else they will break during skewering.
4. Drain and cool.
5. Season the meat with salt and arrange on skewers with the vegetables.
6. In the meantime the salt will have released most of the liquid form the cucumber.
7. Squeeze the remaining liquid from the cucumber; add the mayonnaise and some chopped dill.
8. Brush the skewers with the rosemary oil and grill them for 3 to 4 minutes on a hot grill.
9. Serve with the cucumber salad.

Nutritional values are manually calculated and based on the ingredients specified.
Nutritional value per serving: Calories: 306.1. Fat: 9.1g Saturated Fat: 2.3g Sodium: 1375.0mg. Sugar: 4.4g Carbohydrate 15.8g Protein: 38.2g Dietary fibre: 3.6g

SLOW COOKER CREAMY BEEF STEW WITH ROOT VEGETABLES

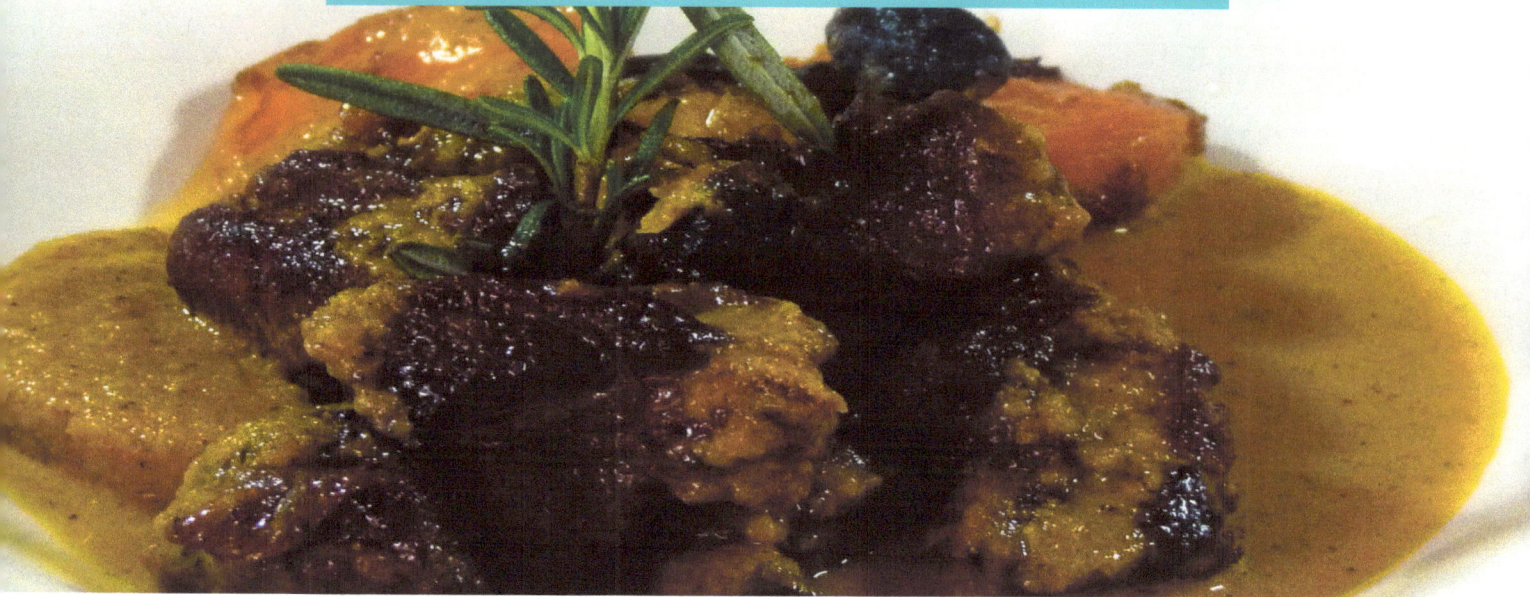

Preparation time: 25 mins

Cooking time: 3 hrs

Total time: 3 hrs 25 mins

When you don't have much time to spend in the kitchen your slow cooker is your best friend! One pot wonders, just place all of the ingredients in the pot and when it is dinner time, the meal is ready. All of the flavours are trapped inside the dish which makes it deliciously intense. For this dish I added a little twist to make the gravy creamier and even more special.

Ingredients: Serves 4

- Small bunch of thyme
- 200gr (6 oz) turnips (cut into wedges)
- 1 large red onion (chopped)
- 2 sprig rosemary • Pink salt • Bone broth
- 125 ml (½ cup) coconut milk

- 200gr (6 oz) carrots (sliced)
- 200gr (6 oz) sweet potato (cut in chunks)
- 3 cloves garlic (sliced)
- 800gr (1 ¾ pound) beef cubes (use some cheaper cuts, shank, brisket or neck)
- 2 fresh bay leaves • 90 ml (3 tbsp) olive oil

Method:

1. Heat the olive oil to high in a large skillet, season the beef with salt, add to the pan and caramelize until well browned.
2. Add the onion, garlic and vegetables, fry for another 2 minutes mixing all ingredients around.
3. Transfer the mix to your slow cooker and top with bone broth until just submerged. Add the herbs and cook for 3 hrs or until the meat is fork tender. Time may vary based on the cut of meat used.
4. When the beef is fork tender transfer the mix to a bowl, separate some of the vegetables and some liquid and place in an upright blender. Add the coconut milk and blend smooth.
5. Divide the beef and balance the vegetables over plates, and finally top with the gravy.

Nutritional values are manually calculated and based on the ingredients specified.
Nutritional value per serving: Calories: 360.9. Fat: 11.5 g. Saturated Fat: 4.5g. Sodium: 221.3 mg. Sugar: 5.7g Carbohydrate 22.5g. Protein: 44.1g. Dietary fibre: 3.9g.

OFFAL

'BISTRO' CHICKEN LIVER PATE WITH VEGETABLE CRACKERS

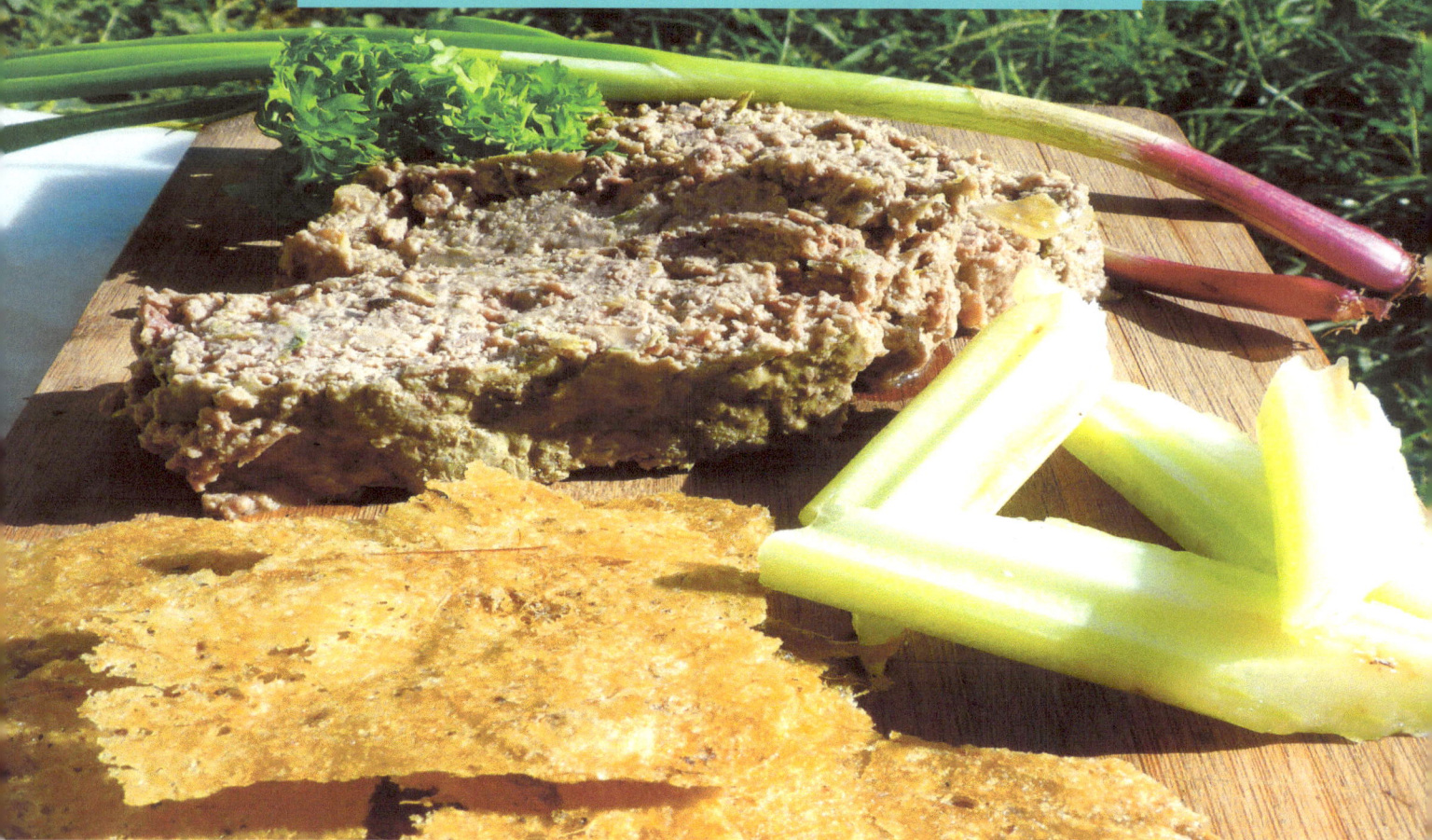

	Preparation time: 20 mins		Cooking time: 40 min for pate 40 min for crackers		Total time: 60min plus chilling time (best chilled overnight)

Crackers I hear you say, on AIP!!?? Yup with a little ingenuity I have created these crackers which are perfect for pate or your favourite dip! A pate is a nutritional powerhouse and also one of my favourite things to snack on, especially with crisp green apple slices! This is a fool proof recipe, super easy to make and the result will surprise you.

Makes one 1.2 kg (2 ¾ pound) loaf

Ingredients: Serves 4

FOR THE PATE:

- 750g (1 ¾ pound) chicken liver
- 150g (5 oz) leeks (sliced small)
- 2 cloves garlic (chopped) • Pink salt

- 450g (1 pound) fatty pork meat (shoulder, belly or minced)
- 1 medium sized onion (cut small)
- 125ml (½ cup) coconut cream

FOR THE CRACKERS:

- 250g (1cup) vegetable pulp
- 50g (1 ¾ tbsp) olive oil
- 20g (1 tsp) garlic powder
- Water

- 120g (4 tbsp) tapioca starch
- 20g (1 tsp) onion powder
- Pink salt

Method:

① If you are using a mincer, cut all of the ingredients until small, and run the veggies through first until well grinded.

② Remove from the bowl, add the pork meat and grind until it looks like mince, do the same with the fat.

③ Remove from the bowl, add the chicken liver and grind. Return the previously grinded ingredients and combine.

④ This is a coarse pate, so you don't have to worry too much about the level of grinding.

⑤ Remove the mix from the bowl; add the coconut cream and fold through, season with salt.

⑥ Place the mix in a baking pan, cover with aluminium foil and bake in a pre-heated oven of 200 degrees (375 F) for about 35 minutes, cooking time depends a bit on the size of your baking pan.

⑦ When you press on the pate it should feel bouncy and firm.

⑧ Allow cooling. When the pate is cooled completely (best overnight) remove from the baking tray by warming the base a bit, the fat in the pate will melt slightly. Turn the baking tray up-side down on a flat surface and the pate will come out.

⑨ Portion the pate; it will last in the fridge for a week or so.

Crackers:

① If you have a juicer, make some vegetable juice like carrot or celery juice, and preserve the pulp. If you don't have a juicer, cut the vegetables into small pieces and grind in a blender, transfer the blended mix to a cheese cloth and strain the juice out, then use the pulp from the cloth.

② Add the starch, onion and garlic powder to the mix plus the oil, mix together until a dough forms. You may need a little water to achieve this, if the pulp is fairly wet you don't need water, but you may need to adjust the starch. You should get a sticky dough.

③ Place the dough on one side of a piece of greased aluminium foil, the size of a baking sheet.

④ Fold the foil over the dough and roll until you have an even sheet of about 3 mm (¼ inches) thickness.

⑤ Bake the sheet in a 160 degree (320 F) oven for 35 minutes or until lightly browned.

⑥ Be careful when touching the foil, it will be very hot, but cools in seconds.

⑦ Open the sheet of foil and remove the crackers carefully. Allow cooling on a rack and break the sheet in cracker size pieces.

Nutritional values are manually calculated and based on the ingredients specified.
(1.2 kg (3 ¾ pounds) batch
Nutritional value per serving: Calories: 4651.9. Fat: 391.0g. Saturated Fat: 138.5g. Sodium: 867.4 mg. Sugar: 9.5g Carbohydrate 33.4g. Protein: 231.8g. Dietary fibre: 4.5g.

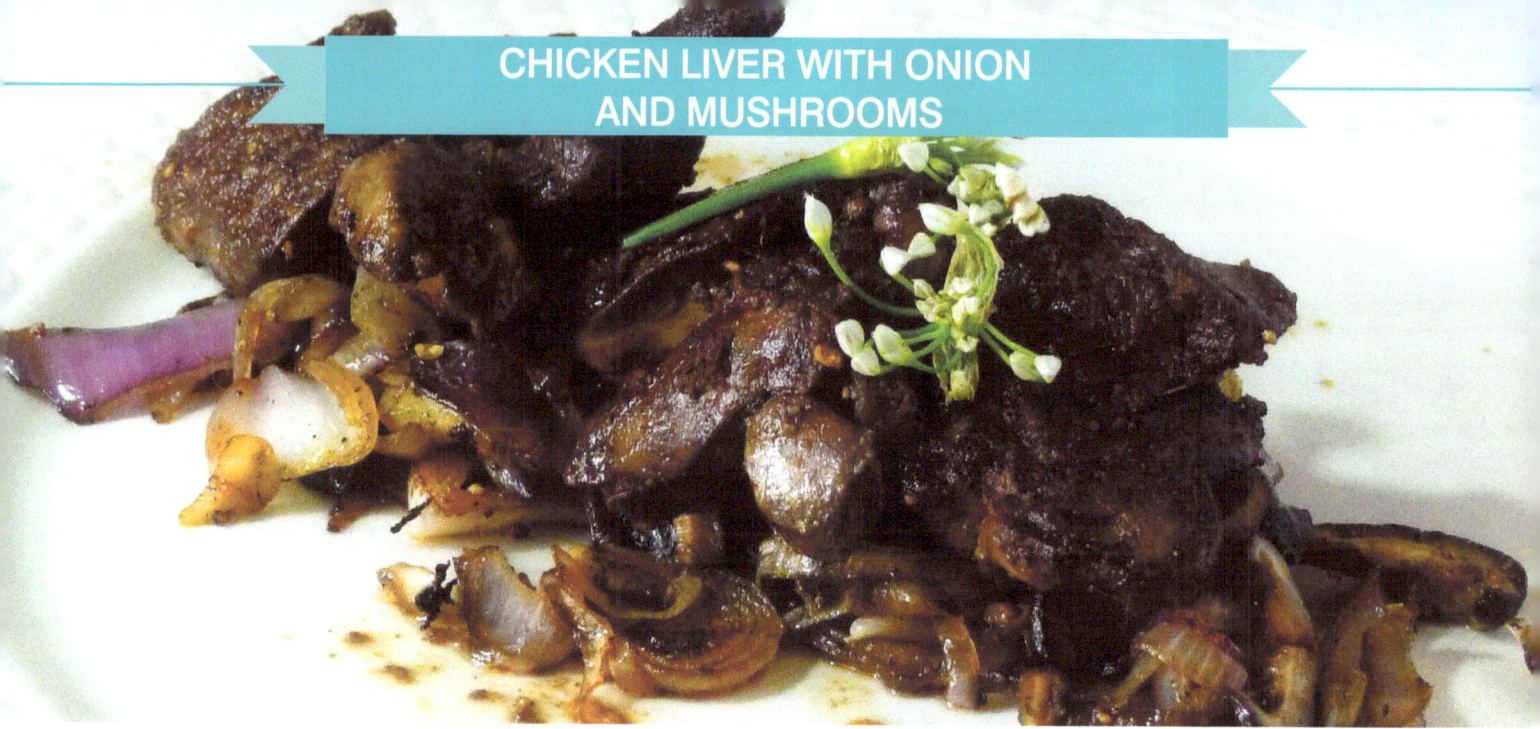

CHICKEN LIVER WITH ONION AND MUSHROOMS

Preparation time: 20 mins

Cooking time: 20 mins

Total time: 40 mins

My Dad made the best livers when I was growing up, the key being not to overcook them so you don't end up with a grainy texture. As I have mentioned offal has key nutrients to aid you on your AIP healing journey, give them a go you may be pleasantly surprised! Crispy fried chicken livers and a good helping of sweet onions and mushrooms completes this dish.

Ingredients: Serves 4

- 600g (1 ½ pound) chicken livers
- 12 button or shi-take mushrooms (sliced)
- 90ml (3 tbsp) olive oil
- Pink salt

- 30g (1 tbsp) tapioca flour
- 450g (1 ½ cups) red onions (sliced)
- 2-3 tsp marjoram

Method:

1. Heat the oil in a skillet to medium heat.
2. Combine the starch with the livers and some salt; fry them until crispy for 3 to 4 minutes and keep aside.
3. Add the onions to the pan and fry for 3 minutes, add the mushrooms and marjoram, fry for another 2 minutes.
4. Place some onion and mushroom mix on plates, arrange the livers on top and drizzle some cooking juice around the dish.

Nutritional values are manually calculated and based on the ingredients specified.
Nutritional value per serving: Calories: 200.4. Fat: 7.5g Saturated Fat: 2.2g Sodium: 103.5mg. Sugar: 0.3g Carbohydrate 8.0g Protein: 25.2g Dietary fibre: 1.3g

LIVER PARFAIT WITH CABBAGE CRACKERS

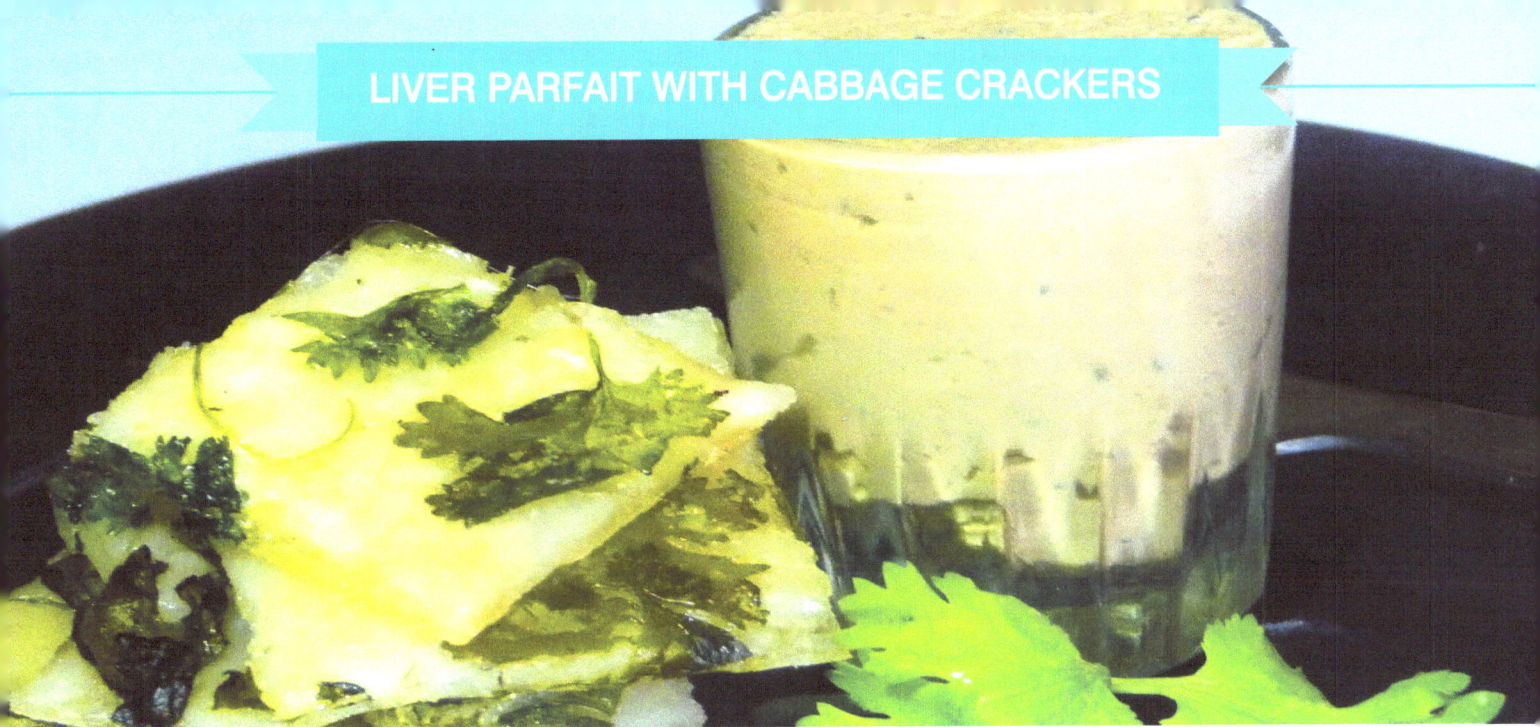

Preparation time:
15 mins

Cooking time:
20 minutes for parfait
35 min for the crackers

Total time:
70 min plus
chilling time

A comfort food for me pre-AIP was creamy liverwurst spread on crusty white bread...Gasp!!! I have recreated the smoothness of liverwurst but this is totally AIP compliant. Making a smooth liver parfait is not as difficult as it sounds; it is delicious and nutritious, therefore worth the effort.

Ingredients: Serves 4

FOR THE PATE:

- 750gr (1 ¾ pound) liver (cut small)

- 15gr (1 tsp) chopped thyme leaves

FOR THE CRACKERS:

- 250gr (1cup) cabbage pulp

- 125 ml (½ cup) coconut cream   • Pink salt

- 50gr (1 ¾ tbsp) olive oil   • 20gr (1 tsp) garlic powder

- Pink salt   • Water

- 120gr (4 tbsp) tapioca starch

- 20gr (1 tsp) onion powder

- 15gr (2 tbsp) coriander leaves

Method:

1. Pre-heat an oven to 150 degrees (300 F).
2. Place the liver, (you can use chicken, pork or beef) with the coconut cream, salt and the thyme in an up-right blender and blend smooth.
3. Transfer the mix to two or three oven proof bowls, place the bowls in a rimmed oven pan.
4. Fill the pan 1/3 with boiling water, cover the bowls with aluminium foil and cook in the oven for 20 to 25 minutes, or until the liver feels firm when touched. Time will vary based on the size of your bowls.
5. When the liver has set remove from the oven and allow chilling in the fridge.
6. When the liver is cold, transfer all to a larger mixing bowl and whisk together to aerate.
7. You will now have a smooth liver parfait.

Nutritional values are manually calculated and based on the ingredients specified.
Nutritional value per serving: Calories: 402.7. Fat: 12.0g. Saturated Fat: 5.4g. Sodium: 205.4 mg. Sugar: 2.6g Carbohydrate 37.2g. Protein: 38.6g. Dietary fibre: 1.2g.

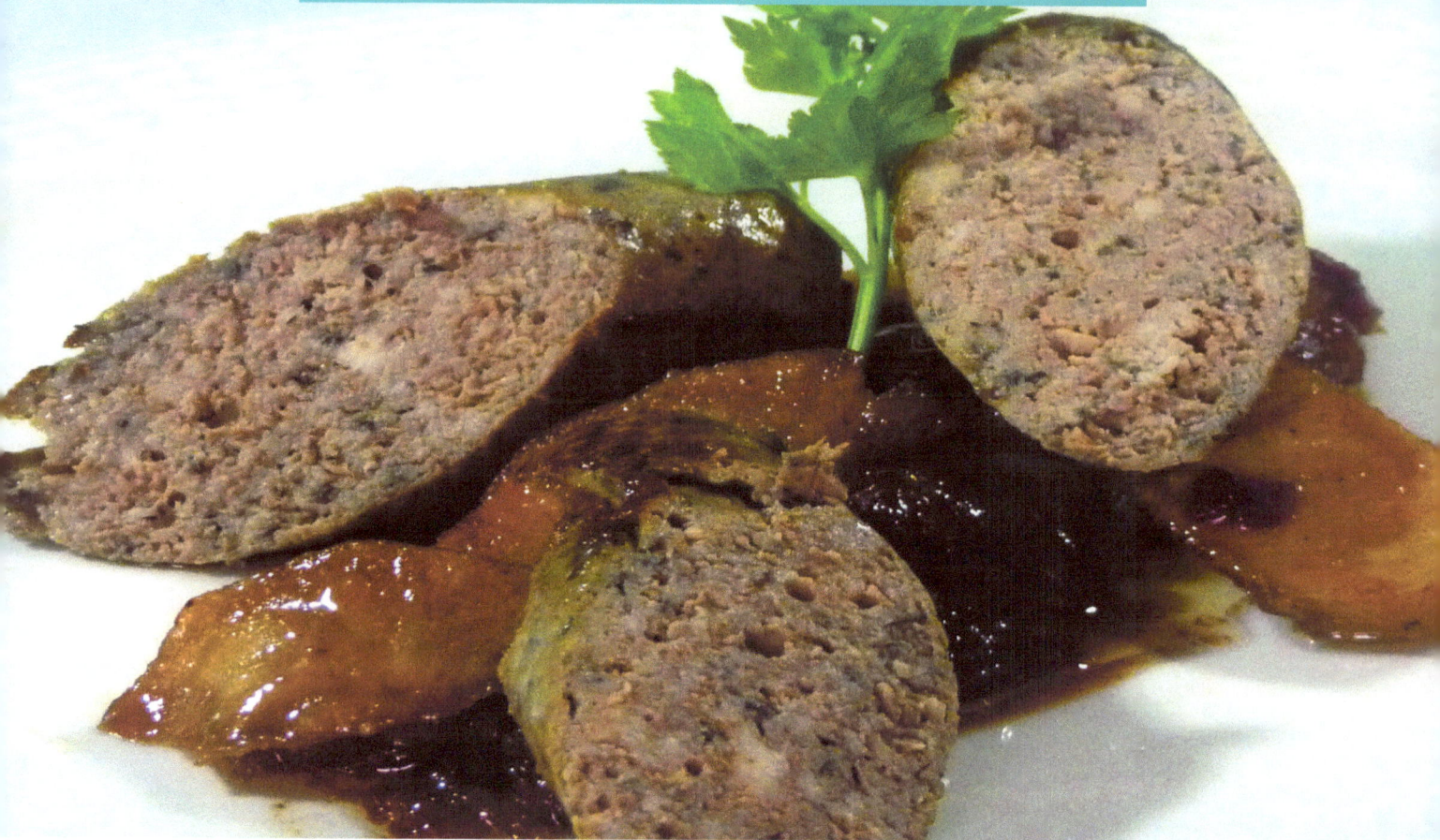

Preparation time:
20 mins

Cooking time:
25 mins

Total time:
45 mins plus
Chilling time

Liver is great offal to make sausages with; you need to add a partly fatty meat to keep them moist. This only increases the quality. Combined with the sweet and sour onion confit, this makes a delicious feast. This is a good dish to make in larger batches and keep in the freezer for later use.

Ingredients:
Serves 4

FOR THE SAUSAGES:

- 600gr (1 ½ pound) pork liver
- 1 medium onion (finely chopped)
- 5gr (½ tsp) ground sage
- 60ml (2 tbsp) olive oil

- 250gr (8 oz) fatty pork meat (minced, neck or blade steak)
- 2 cloves garlic (chopped)
- 5gr (½ tsp) marjoram
- Pink salt

FOR THE CONFIT:

- 500gr (2 cups) red onions (sliced)
- 60 ml (2 tbsp) vinegar
- 60 ml (2 tbsp) olive oil

- 1 large apple (cored, peeled and sliced in thin wedges)
- 30gr (1 tbsp) coconut sugar

Method:

1. Cut the liver and the pork meat into small pieces, place in a food processor and blend into a fine, slight course mix.

2. Add the herbs, onion, garlic and some salt, pulse to combine.
   Spread a piece of cling wrap on a flat surface and spread 1/8 of the mix, about 120gr (4 oz) over the sheet.

3. Roll the mix into a 12 cm (5 inch) long sausage shape and tie a knot on both ends so the sausage is tightly secured.

4. Fill a flat braising pan with enough water to cover the sausages.

5. Bring the water to about 80 degrees (175 F) add the sausages and cook for 10 minutes.

6. Turn off the heat and allow the sausages to cool in the water.

7. Remove the sausages from the water and cool completely; best overnight.

8. Meanwhile make the onion confit.

9. Heat the oil to low medium heat, frying the onion slices in the oil on low heat until they start to soften and brown. Add the apple, sugar and continue to fry for another 2 minutes.

10. Add the vinegar and cook another 5 minutes, allow cooling time.

11. Remove the sausages from the cling wrap when they are fully chilled through.

12. Heat the oil in a skillet to medium high and fry the sausages for 2 to 3 minutes.

13. Serve with the apple onion confit.

Nutritional values are manually calculated and based on the ingredients specified.
Nutritional value per serving: Calories: 473.8 Fat: 27.4g Saturated Fat: 6.5g Sodium: 40.1mg.
Sugar: 3.0g Carbohydrate 13.6g Protein: 43.4g Dietary fibre: 2.3g

OX- TONGUE WITH SALSA VERDE, RAISINS, CAPERS AND SWEET POTATO

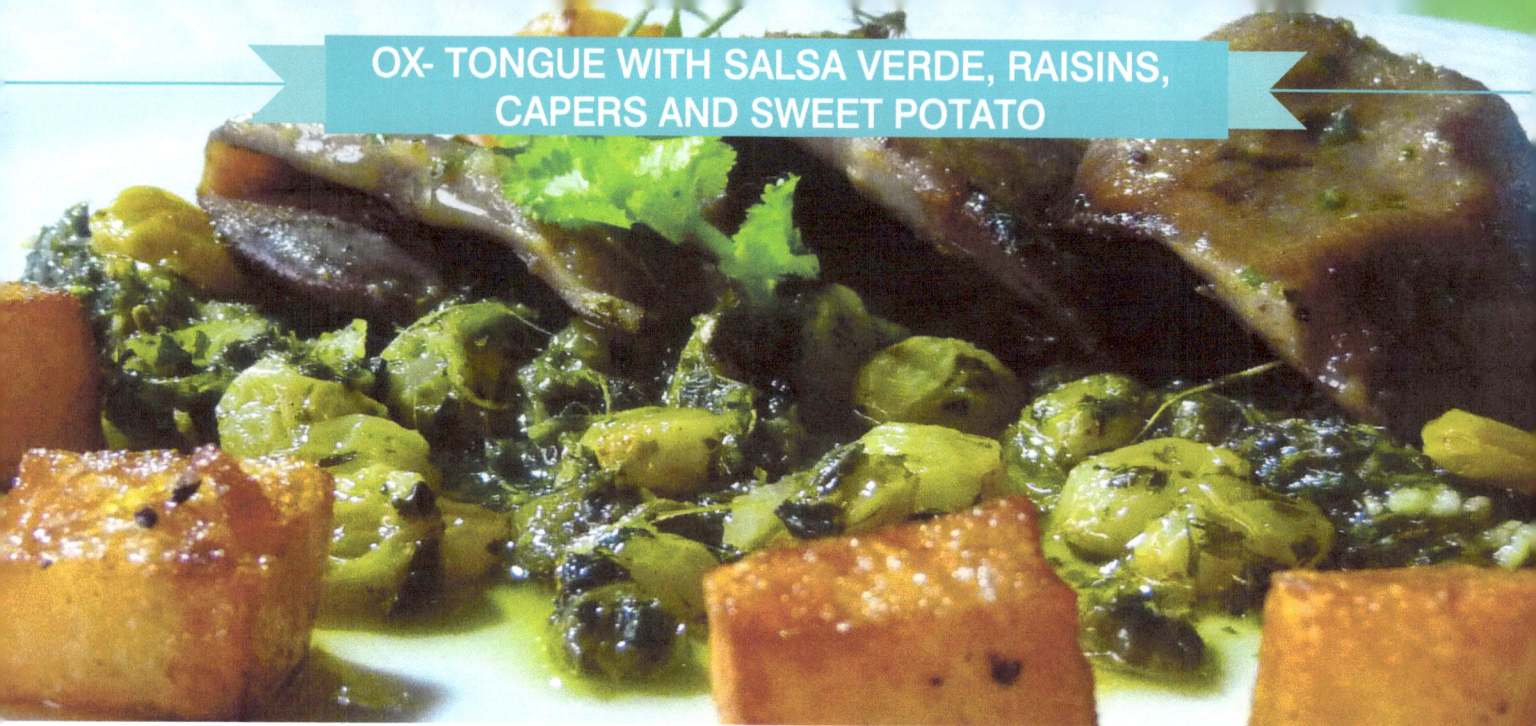

Preparation time: 25 mins		Cooking time: 1 hr 10 mins		Total time: 1 hr 35 mins	

Ox-tongue is one piece of offal meat that is often overlooked, however it is a must try. Brawn is a real delicacy made mostly with pressed tongue and often a special treat for me when I visit the butchers. This is a new way to introduce offal to your AIP diet.

Ingredients: Serves 4

* 600gr (1 ½ pound) ox-tongue (without throat)
* 25gr (4 tbsp) fresh coriander leaves
* 1 small onion (roughly cut)   *   Pink salt
* Juice of ½ lime   *   40gr (1 ½ tbsp) capers
* 450gr (1 pound) sweet potatoes (cut into generous cubes)

* 60 ml (2 tbsp) olive oil
* 25gr (4 tbsp) sage leaves
* 2 cloves garlic (crushed)
* 125ml (½ cup) olive oil   *   Oil or fat of choice for frying
* 90gr (3 tbsp) golden raisins

Method:

1. Place the ox-tongue in a stockpot, submerge with water and bring to a boil. Lower the heat and simmer for 1 to 1 ½ hours. The time will depend on the size of the tongue, when the skin peels off easily the tongue is cooked. Allow cooling in the water.
2. Meanwhile place the herbs with the onion, a little salt and garlic in an up-right blender, add the lime juice and blend in. With the blender running add the 125 ml oil.
3. When the tongue has cooled down enough to handle by hand, peel the skin off and discard. Slice the tongue at a 45 degree angle in thin slices.
4. Heat the oil for frying to 180 degrees (350 F) and fry the sweet potato cubes golden and crisp, for 3 to 4 minutes.
5. Heat the two tbsp olive oil in a skillet and fry the tongue slices for a few seconds on both sides. Remove from the pan and keep aside.
6. Add the salsa verde to the pan with the capers and raisins, mix well.
7. Divide the salsa verde over plates, top with slices of ox-tongue and surround with sweet potato cubes.

Nutritional values are manually calculated and based on the ingredients specified.
Nutritional value per serving: Calories: 633.4. Fat: 38.2g. Saturated Fat: 12.5g. Sodium: 469.5mg. Sugar: 13.3g Carbohydrate 46.6g. Protein: 24.8g. Dietary fibre: 4.8g.

POACHED CHICKEN SALAD WITH FRIED CHICKEN LIVER

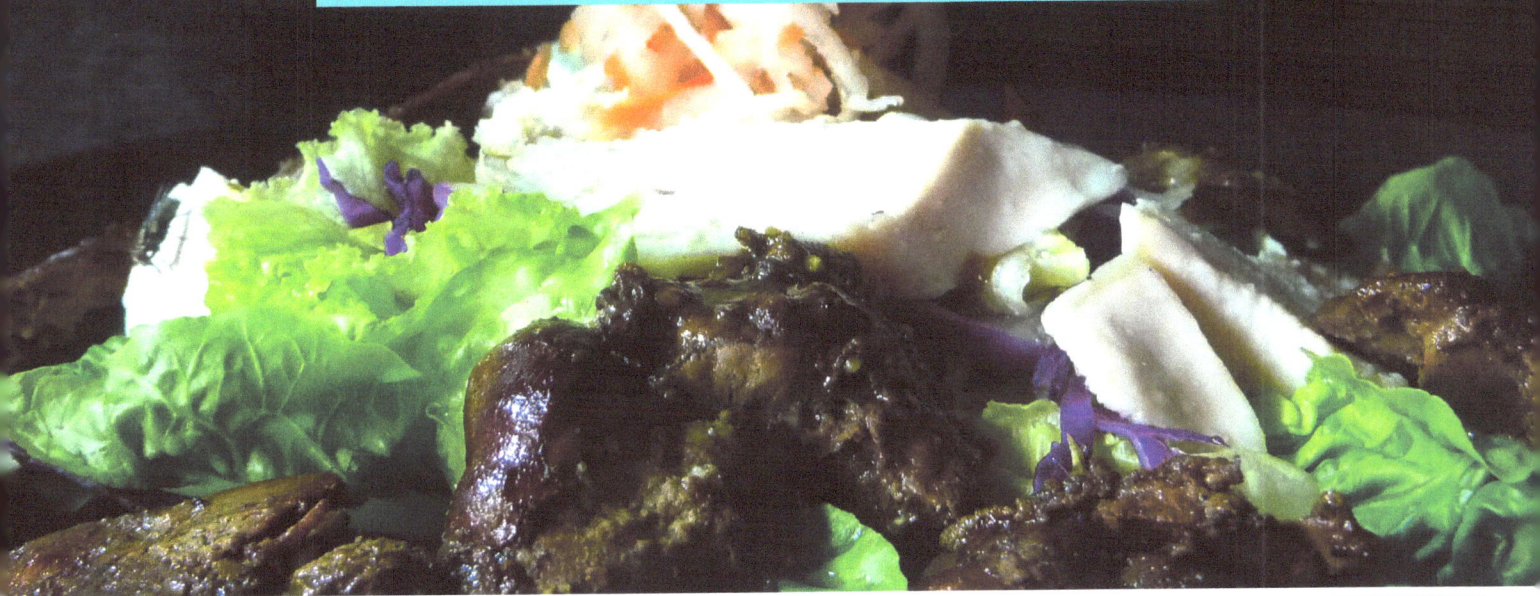

Preparation time: 15 mins

Cooking time: 45 mins

Total time: 60 mins

When we talk about chicken salad we usually imagine left over roasted chicken being used, often somewhat dry and chewy. Poaching will keep the chicken soft and moist, which makes it a delight for the palate. I have added fried chicken livers for contrast in taste and added nutrition. The combination is a concoction not to be denied!

Ingredients: Serves 4

- 350gr (12 oz) chicken breast
- 250ml (1 cup) chicken broth
- 120gr (4 oz) shredded carrot
- 1 medium sized onion (sliced)
- Juice of ½ a lime   •   Pink salt

- 15gr (1 tsp) dried thyme
- 350gr (12oz) chicken liver
- 120gr (4 oz) shredded radish
- 90 ml (3 tbsp) olive oil
- Mixed salad leaves

Method:

1. Season the chicken breast with salt and rub the dried thyme all over the breasts.
2. Place the breast in a saucepan, add the chicken broth and turn on the heat. When the broth just comes to a boil, lower the heat and let the breasts cook through, just below boiling point. This takes about 3 to 4 minutes, ensure not to overcook the breast. Allow cooling in the broth.
3. Meanwhile pre-heat an oven to 180 degrees (350 F), place the chicken liver on an oven tray, sprinkle a little salt and 30 ml (1 tbsp) of the oil over them. Bake for ten minutes.
4. Combine the remaining oil with the lime juice.
5. When the livers have baked for ten minutes, heat a skillet to high heat and transfer the livers to the skillet. Fry them for 30 seconds to 1 minute, until crisp. Remove from the pan and add the dressing to the pan. The dressing will deglaze the pan in a few seconds, turn off the heat.
6. Arrange the salad leaves on plates, top with shredded carrot and radish.
7. Slice the chicken breast in ½ cm (¼ inch) thick slices and arrange on the salad, lastly add the livers and drizzle the dressing over the dish.
8. Serve slightly warm.

Nutritional values are manually calculated and based on the ingredients specified.
Nutritional value per serving: Calories: 313.6 Fat: 17.5g Saturated Fat: 3.9g Sodium: 118.4mg. Sugar: 1.2g Carbohydrate 3.4g Protein: 34.5g Dietary fibre: 1.5g

PORK RIB AND PORK TAIL STEW

Preparation time: 15 mins

Cooking time: 1 hr 30 mins

Total time: 1 hr 45 mins

Paleo and AIP lifestyles are all about respect for the animals we consume, and a big part of this is the nose to tail philosophy. If you are a stew person and hearty meals are on your list of favourites, then this is a must try recipe. Ox tail may be better known to many, but pork tail is second to none. This dish works well in a slow cooker as well. Just transfer all ingredients after frying to your slow cooker and cook on low for 4 to 5 hours.

Ingredients: Serves 4

- 450gr (1 pound) pork back ribs
- 1 medium sized carrot (cut in chunky pieces)
- 125gr (½ cup) turnip (cut in chunky pieces)
- 2 cloves garlic (crushed)
- 2 sprig rosemary • Pink salt
- 60 ml (2 tbsp) olive oil

- 500 ml (2 cups) bone broth
- 450gr (1 pound) pork tail
- 2 stalks celery (cut in 3 cm, 1 inch pieces)
- 1 medium sized onion (cut into wedges)
- Small bunch of thyme
- 1-2 fresh bay leaves

Method:

1. Heat the oil in a skillet to medium heat; add the ribs and the pork tail and fry them brown, for about 5 minutes.
2. When they are browned add all of the vegetables and fry for another 2 minutes. While stirring all of the ingredients around add a little salt while doing so.
3. Add the bone broth, thyme and rosemary, lower the heat, cover the pan and simmer for 1 ½ hours. Time may vary depending on the size of the meat. Adjust the liquid when necessary.
4. Remove the meat from the pot, allow it to cool for a little while, divide into 4 equal portions.
5. Serve the dish with the vegetables, some broth and mashed sweet potatoes.

Nutritional values are manually calculated and based on the ingredients specified.
Nutritional value per serving: Calories: 1012.4. Fat: 75.5g Saturated Fat: 24.6g, Sodium: 375.9mg. Sugar: 3.6g Carbohydrate 22.8g. Protein: 58.9g. Dietary fibre: 3.8g.

VEGETABLE CONFETTI WITH PORK LIVER, ONION RINGS AND CRISPY PROSCIUTTO

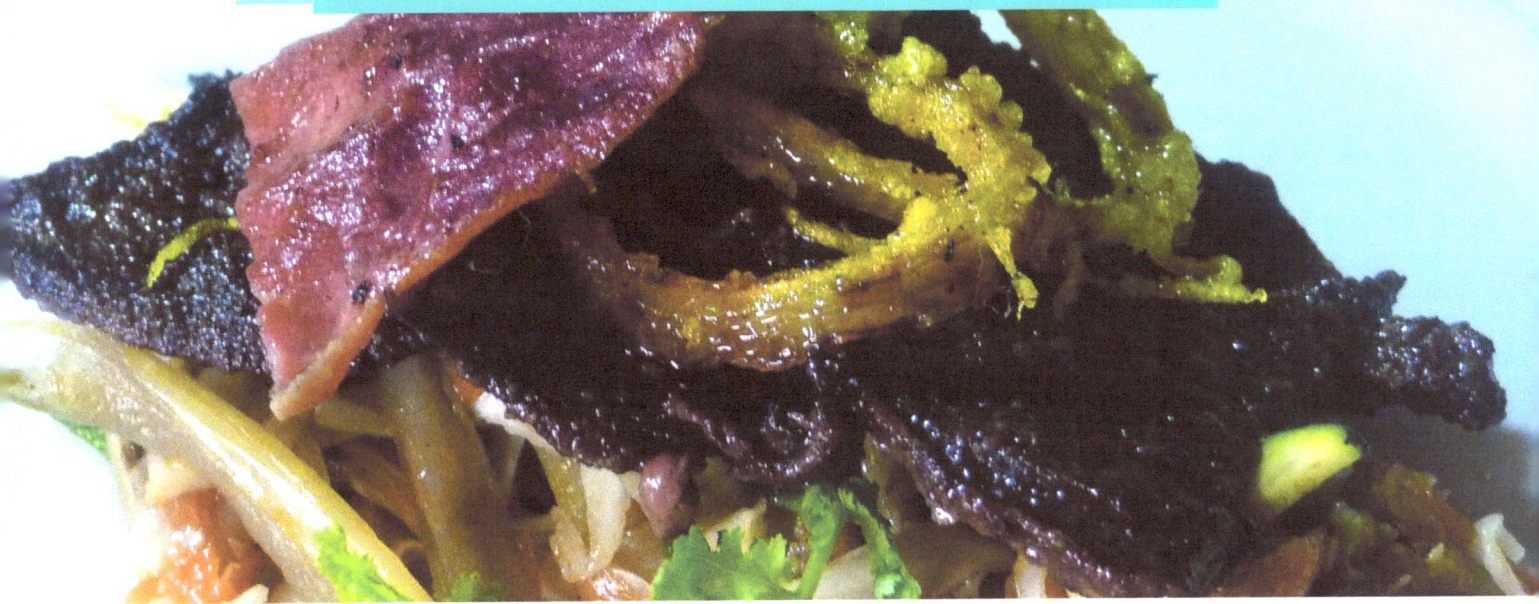

Preparation time: 25 mins

Cooking time: 15 mins

Total time: 40 mins

Offal used to be an integral part of our diets but, as our view of food has changed over the decades, it has sadly all but disappeared from our plates. A lot of people have been turned off by offal because of a bad food experience or even just the idea of what it is. When cooked correctly it really is delicious! Offal meat is rich in vitamins, easy to prepare, delicious and cheap!

Ingredients:

Serves 4

FOR THE VEGETABLES:

- 800gr (2 pounds) mixed vegetables to your liking (I used carrot, fennel, celery, cabbage, zucchini and turnip)
- 90gr (3 tbsp) tapioca flour
- 60 ml (2 tbsp) olive oil
- Sea salt

FOR THE LIVER:

- 650gr (1 ½ pound) pork liver (thinly sliced)

- 12 onion rings
- 5gr (½ tsp) turmeric powder
- Oil for frying
- 60gr (2 tbsp) tapioca flour
- Pink salt
- 2 slices prosciutto

Method:

1. Cut all of the vegetables into fine strips, the idea is to get a colourful mix.
2. Combine the tapioca flour with the turmeric. Add some water so that you get a light batter.
3. Season the pork liver with a little salt and dust in the tapioca flour.
4. Heat some oil for frying (in a deep fryer at 180 degrees, 350 F, or about 2 cm, 3/4 inch deep in a skillet). Dip the onion rings in the batter and fry them for about 3 minutes until golden and crisp.
5. Meanwhile, heat a skillet with the olive oil to medium heat. Fry the liver for 1 to 2 minutes on both sides, depending on the thickness of the slices. Don't fry for too long or the liver will become very dry. It should be slightly pink in the middle.
6. Remove from the pan and keep aside. Add the prosciutto slices to the pan and fry them until crisp.
7. Add the olive oil from the vegetables to the pan and turn the heat to high. When the oil is smoking hot add the vegetables and stir-fry for 2 minutes until cooked, and still crunchy. Check for taste.
8. Divide the vegetables over 4 plates, top with the onion rings and half a slice of the prosciutto.
9. Serve hot.

Nutritional values are manually calculated and based on the ingredients specified.
Nutritional value per serving: Calories: 415.4. Fat: 20.0g. Saturated Fat: 4.1g. Sodium: 352.7 mg. Sugar: 6.1g Carbohydrate 19.6g. Protein: 39.9g. Dietary fibre: 3.6 g.

DESSERTS

COCONUT PANNA COTTA WITH FRUIT

Preparation time: 15 mins

Cooking time: 10 mins

Total time: 25 mins plus Chilling time

When I was working at Vine Restaurant Mimma's Panna Cotta was one of my absolute favourite desserts, and it was also a firm favourite amongst the loyal clientele! Panna Cotta is such a traditional dish, beloved all over Italy and in many other parts of the world. I have recreated the silky creaminess that we all know and love in a good Panna Cotta without the dairy. A beautiful guilt free treat!

Ingredients:
Serves 4

- 4 cups coconut cream
- 2 tsp vanilla powder
- 6 tbsp cold water
- ¼ cup water • 2 tbsp Coconut sugar

- 1/4 cup Coconut sugar
- 4 ½ tsp agar-agar powder
- 1 cup cherries (or any other fruit to your liking) de-stoned
- 1 tbsp lemon juice

Method:

1. Combine the agar-agar powder with the water.
2. Heat the coconut cream with the sugar in a saucepan. Once the sugar is dissolved, add the agar-agar ensuring a soft boil.
3. Remove from the heat and stir in the vanilla powder.
4. Ladle the mix in individual serving bowls, if you use glasses allow a little cooling to ensure the glasses can withstand the heat.
5. Allow to cool completely.
6. Chop the cherries up finely and lace with the water, lemon juice and sugar in a sauce pan.
7. Bring to boil, lower the heat and simmer for 5 minutes or until the mixture thickens and becomes pulpy.
8. Allow to cool before use.
9. Serve the Panna Cotta chilled with the warm or cold fruit coulis and top with fruit of your choice.

Nutritional values are manually calculated and based on the ingredients specified.
Nutritional value per serving: Calories: 219.4 Fat: 5.1g. Saturated Fat: 5.0g. Sodium: 30.6mg Sugar: 18.0g Carbohydrate 43.7g. Protein: 1.4g. Dietary fibre: 0.6g.

COCONUT BANANA FLAN WITH FRUIT COMPOTE

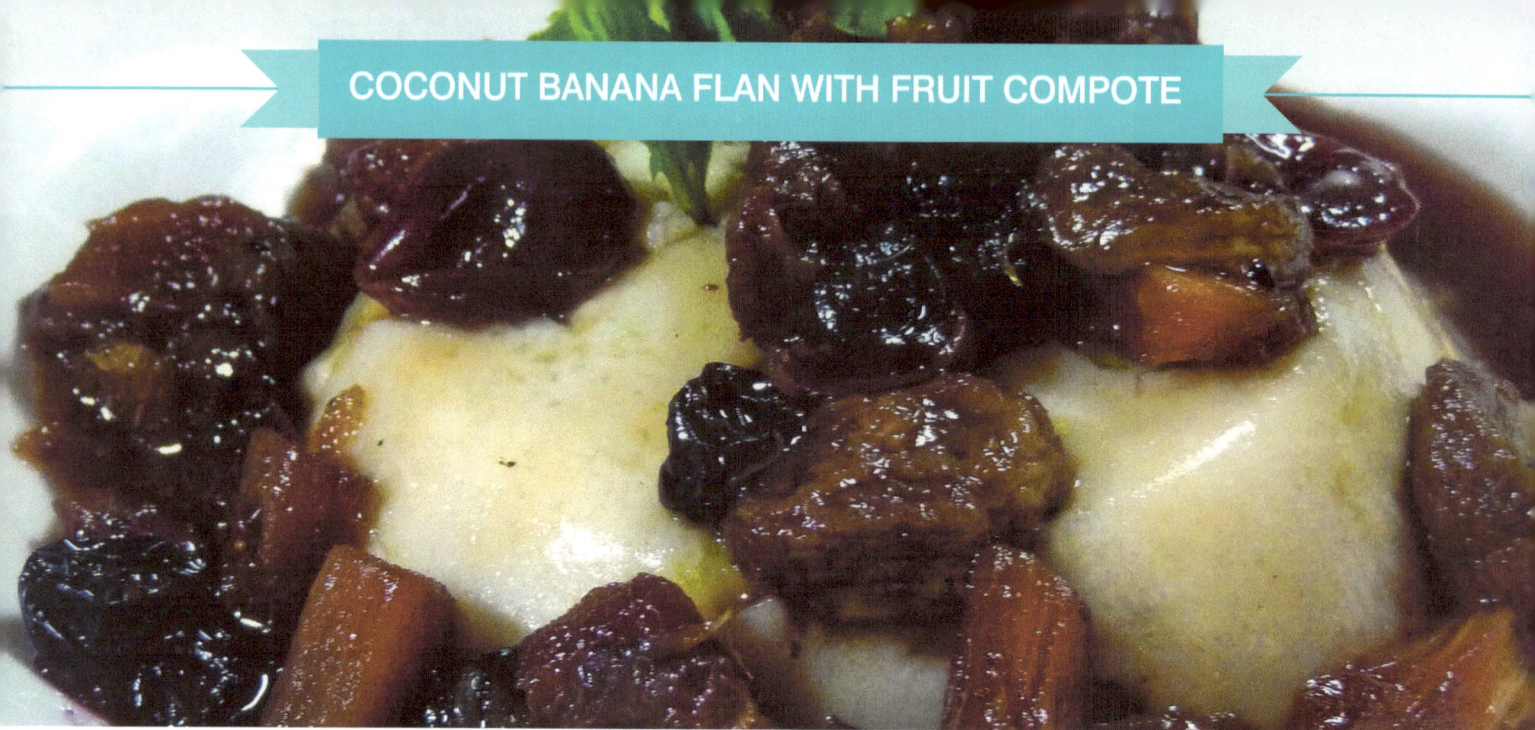

Preparation time: 15 mins

Cooking time: 10 mins

Total time: 25 mins plus Chilling time

Just because you are doing AIP doesn't mean you can't indulge in a little sweet affair every now and then! This is a beautiful creamy, light dessert that will make you want to make a double batch next time. Experiment with your favourite stone fruits, berries or even stewed apple or pear for the middle of the flan and play around with the components of the compote, create your own unique signature!! Tip: be wary of using pineapple or kiwi fruit when making desserts with gelatin as the enzymes in these fruits will inhibit the gelatin from setting.

Ingredients: Serves 4

- 650 ml (2 ¾ cup) coconut milk
- 30gr (2 tbsp) mint leaves (chopped)
- 400gr (1 ½ cup) mixed fruit (berries, pineapple, grapes, kiwi fruit)
- 1 small cinnamon stick

- 4 small bananas
- 30 ml (1 tbsp) vanilla powder
- Juice of 1 lime
- 8gr (2tspn) grass fed gelatine granules

Method:

1. Bring the coconut milk to a soft boil with the mint and vanilla powder. Add the gelatin and ladle a small layer on the bases of 4 individual bowls. Ensure the bowls are wet before doing this which will allow easy removal of the flan from the bowls. Let this firm up for 20 minutes or so in the fridge.
2. Cut the bananas lengthwise in half, then in quarters and then crosswise in small pieces.
3. When the base layers have firmed up a bit, divide the bananas over the bowls. The base will prevent the banana pieces from sinking through the base (later the top) of the flan.
4. Divide the remaining coconut over the bowls and chill.
5. Meanwhile cut the fruit used for the compote where needed and add with the sugar, cinnamon, lime juice and a little water to a small sauce pan.
6. Bring to a soft boil and simmer for 10 minutes, allow cooling.
7. Carefully loosen the sides of the flan with a small knife and turn the bowls up-side down on plates, shake a bit and the flan should come out of the bowls.
8. Top with the fruit compote and serve.

> **Nutritional values are manually calculated and based on the ingredients specified.**
> **Nutritional value per serving:** Calories: 177.2 Fat: 3.8g Saturated Fat: 3.2g Sodium: 20.6mg. Sugar: 18.2g Carbohydrate 36.7 g Protein: 2.1 g Dietary fibre: 4.4g

COCONUT ICE CREAM

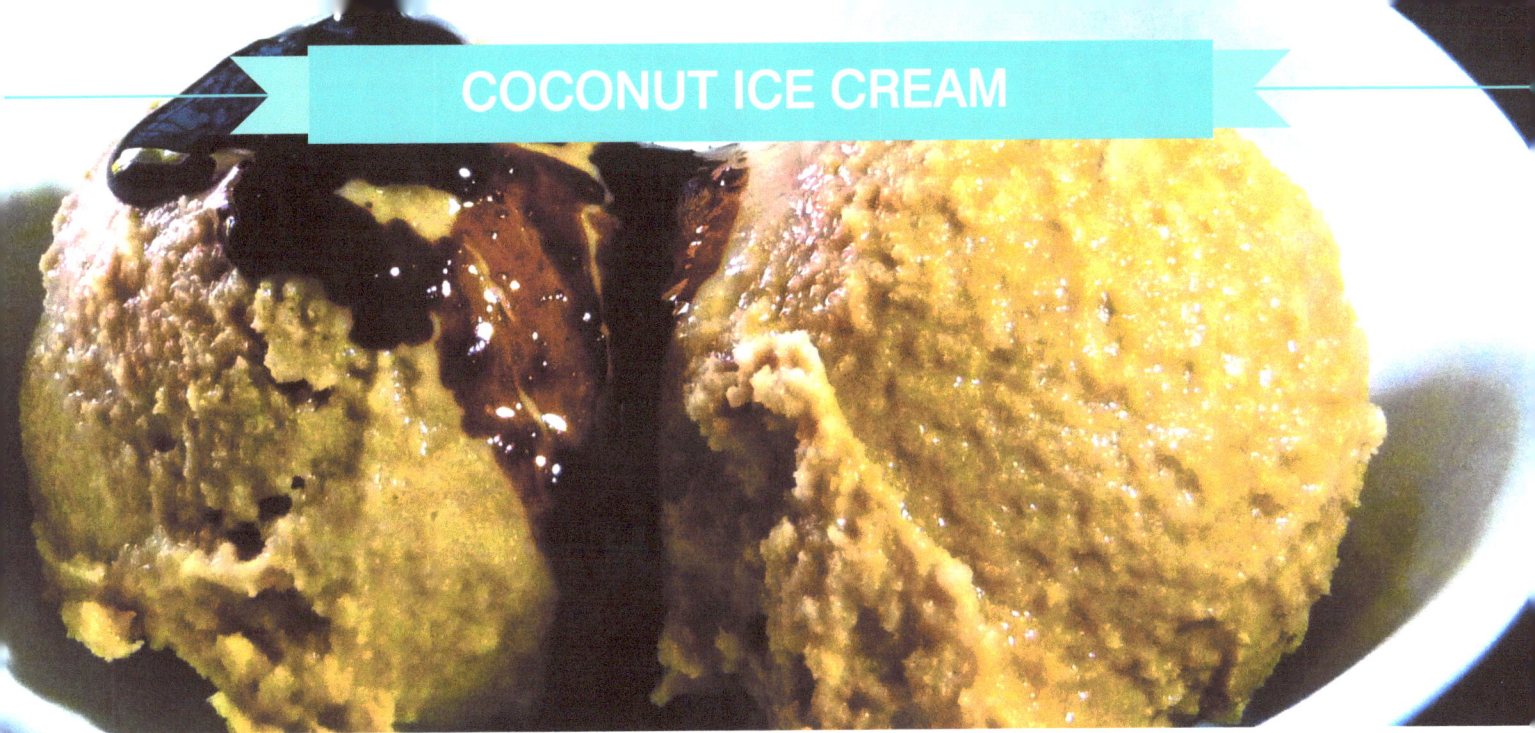

Preparation time:
15 mins

Total time:
15 mins plus chilling time

I scream, you scream, we all scream for ice cream!! This super simple ice cream recipe is a perfect base for you to go wild and experiment with your favourite AIP flavours! Delicious as is, or try something extra like a teaspoon of peppermint extract or even fresh mint or mixing in some chopped berries. You will get a much smoother result if you have an ice cream maker however you can still get a good result without one. Keep in mind that homemade ice cream sets very hard compared to store bought ice creams, because of the lack of thickeners and emulsifiers, used in commercial ice creams. All you have to do is set it out on the bench for a while to soften.

Ingredients: Serves 4

- 700 ml (24 oz) coconut milk

- 30 ml (2 tsp) vanilla powder

- 1 ripe avocado

- 150 ml (5 oz) maple syrup

- Pinch of pink salt

Method:

1. Blend the coconut, maple syrup, avocado and vanilla powder together in an upright blender and place in your ice cream maker. Follow the instructions that come with the machine.
2. If you don't have one, place the mix in a covered container and place in the freezer, mix every hour or so until frozen.
3. If you have other things to do and you find a hard frozen block in the freezer when you check it, just allow it to defrost a bit, break in to small pieces and pulse smooth in a food processor.
4. Serve with a drizzle of maple syrup or fruit of your choice.

Nutritional values are manually calculated and based on the ingredients specified.
Nutritional value per serving: Calories: 121.5 Fat: 1.3g Saturated Fat: 1.1g, Sodium: 7.6mg. Sugar: 18.1g Carbohydrate 28.6g Protein: 1.1g Dietary fibre: 2.3g

COCONUT PUDDING WITH BERRIES

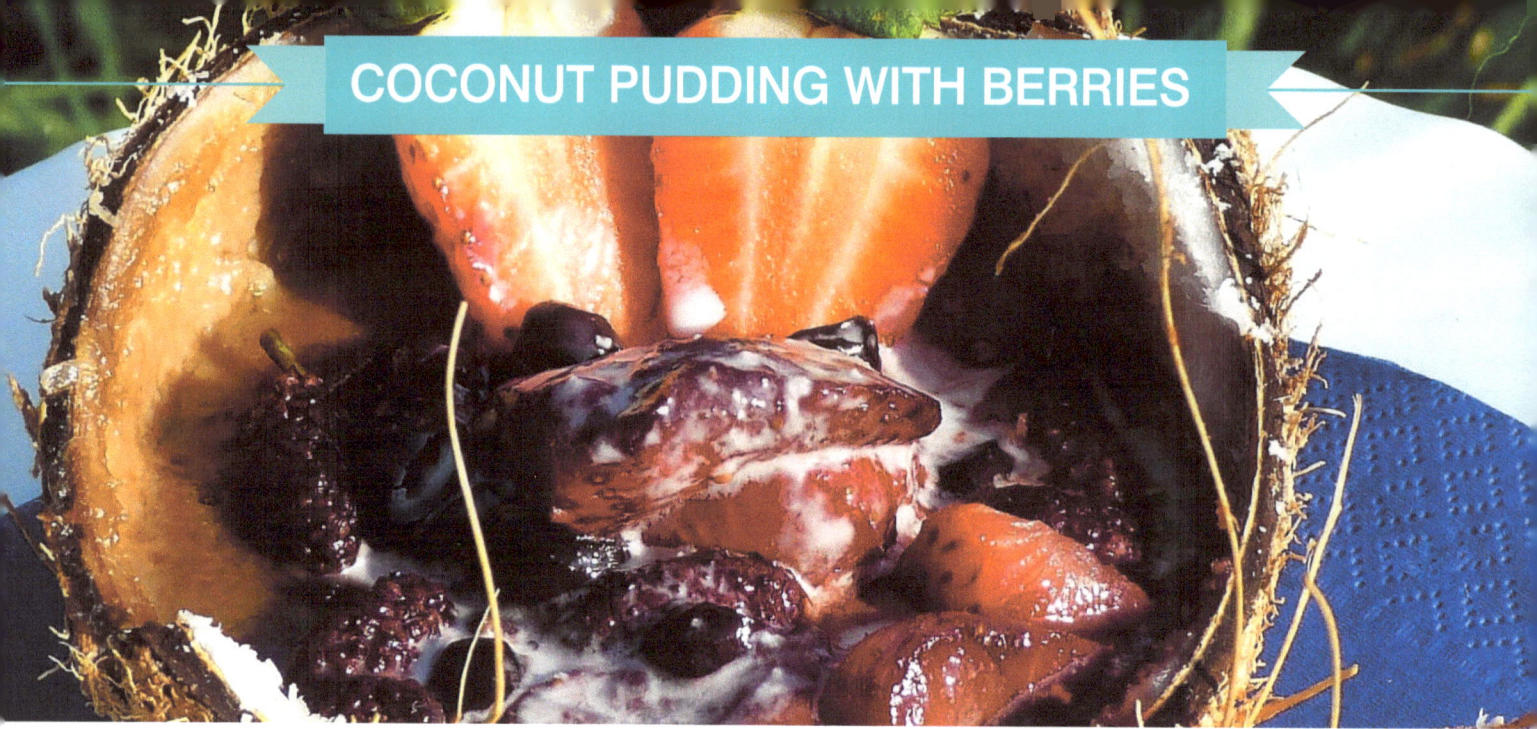

Preparation time:
15 mins

Cooking time:
05 mins

Total time:
20 mins plus
Cooking time

"If you don't eat your vegetables, you can't have any pudding" is a saying that appeared on a Pink Floyd album if I am not mistaken! For this pudding you will eat any vegetables, believe me. A lovely sweet, smooth coconut pudding is combined with delicious berries - Simply irresistible.

Ingredients: Serves 4

FOR THE PUDDING:

♦ 600ml (1.2pnt) coconut milk

♦ 8g (¼ oz) gelatine

FOR THE BERRIES:

♦ 12 strawberries (cut in half)

♦ 40g (2 oz) mulberries

♦ 45g (1 1/2oz) coconut sugar

♦ Zest of half a lemon

♦ 40g (2 oz) blueberries

♦ 10g (1 tbsp) chopped mint leaves

♦ 40ml (1 ½ oz) maple syrup

Method:

① Bring the coconut milk with the sugar and the lemon zest to a soft boil. Add the gelatin, when the coconut milk starts to boil again, remove from the heat and divide over 4 serving bowls. Allow cooling.

② Meanwhile place the berries with the maple syrup and a little water in a small sauce pan.

③ Bring to a simmer and cook for 5 minutes so the fruit has softened and the liquid has thickened.

④ Top the pudding with the berry compote and serve with a drizzle of coconut milk or coyo.

Nutritional values are manually calculated and based on the ingredients specified.
Nutritional value per serving: Calories: 121.5 Fat: 1.3g Saturated Fat: 1.1g, Sodium: 7.6mg. Sugar: 18.1g Carbohydrate 28.6g Protein: 1.1g Dietary fibre: 2.3g

FRUIT SOUP

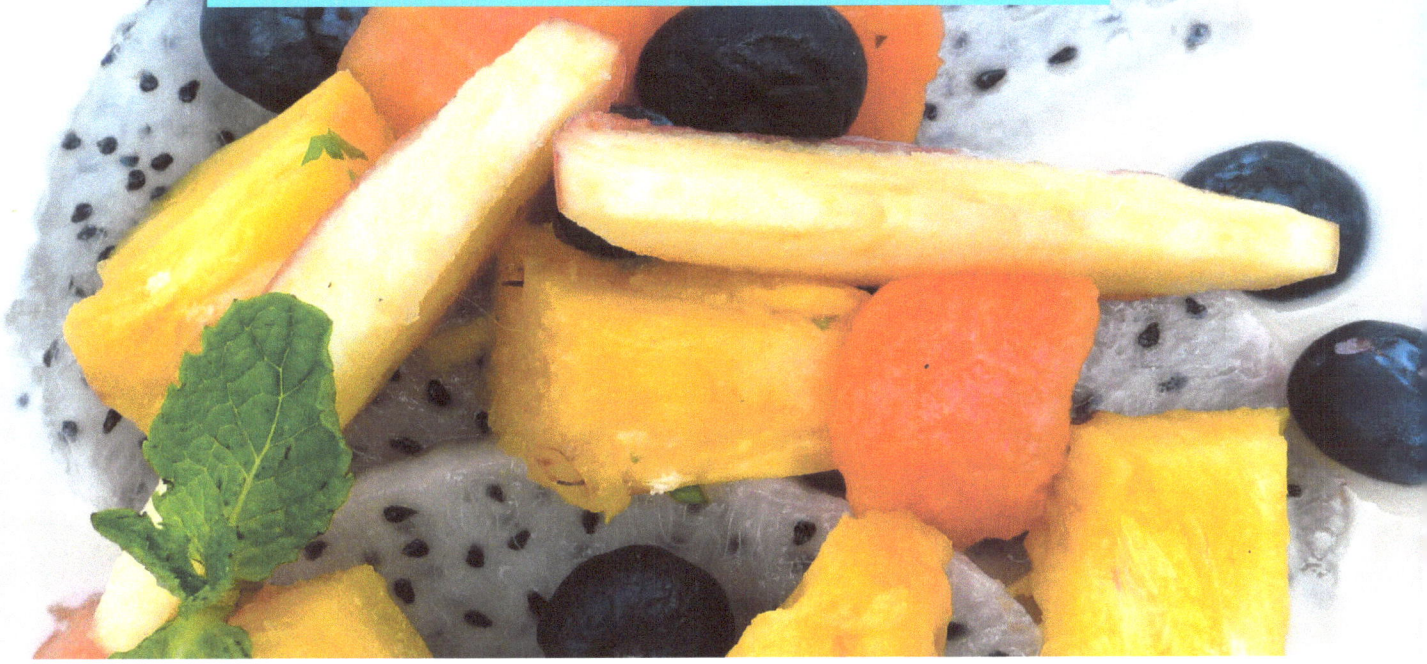

Preparation time:
10 mins

Cooking time:
20 mins

Total time:
30 mins plus
Cooking time

Need a quick dessert in a pinch, or an indulgent weekend brunch? This coconut fruit soup is easily adaptable to whatever fruit you have on hand, however if you have never tried dragon fruit do yourself a favour and give it a try. It is a very smooth silky textured fruit that works amazingly in this coconut soup.

Ingredients: Serves 4

- 600 ml (20 fl oz) coconut milk

- 90 ml (3 tbsp) maple syrup

- 400 g (13 oz) of any fruit
  (cut into bite size pieces)

- 1 tbsp grass fed gelatin granules

- 15g (1 tbsp) chopped mint leaves

Method:

1. Bring the coconut milk and gelatin, with the maple syrup and the mint leaves, to a soft boil. If you use fresh coconut milk you will see that the coconut milk splits, place the mix in an up-right blender and pulse for a few seconds and your soup will be perfect.

2. If you use UHT coconut milk, this may not happen, if it does, follow the same procedure.
3. Place some fruit in deep plates and poor the soup around the fruit.

4. Serve at room temperature or chilled.

Nutritional values are manually calculated and based on the ingredients specified.
Nutritional value per serving: Calories: 126.9. Fat: 3.7 g Saturated Fat: 2.8 g   Sodium: 18.8 mg. Sugar: 21.1 g
Carbohydrate 24.8 g Protein: 14.9 g Dietary fibre: 1.1 g

FRUITY GRANITA

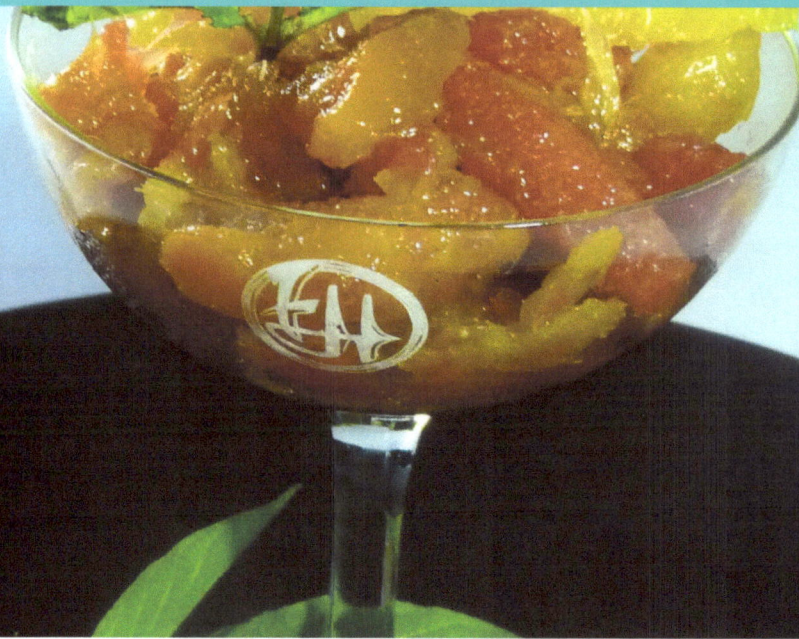

Preparation time:
15 mins

Total time:
15 mins plus
8 hrs Freezing time

Granitas are a very simple dessert and are also a perfect way to cool down on a hot summer afternoon. Another recipe for you that you can play around with and choose your favourite combinations! There's nothing much to it, mix, freeze and scrape. They are refreshing, healthy and so good!

Ingredients:
Serves 4

- 900gr (2 pounds) of any fruit, I used orange and grapefruit

- 250gr (1 cup) fruit juice

- Juice of ½ a lemon

- 30gr (1 tbsp) maple syrup

Method:

1. Clean the fruit you use and chop into small pieces.

2. Combine the fruit with the fruit juice, lemon juice and maple syrup.

3. Place the mix into a shallow baking tray that will fit in your freezer. Freeze for about 8 hours, when the mix has hardened scrape with a fork over the surface so you get a shaved ice effect.

4. Transfer to serving bowls or glasses and serve immediately.

Nutritional values are manually calculated and based on the ingredients specified.
Nutritional value per serving: Calories: 59.2 Fat: 0.1g Saturated Fat: 0.0g. Sodium: 0.0 mg. Sugar: 12.7g Carbohydrate 14.9g Protein: 1.1g Dietary fibre: 2.5g

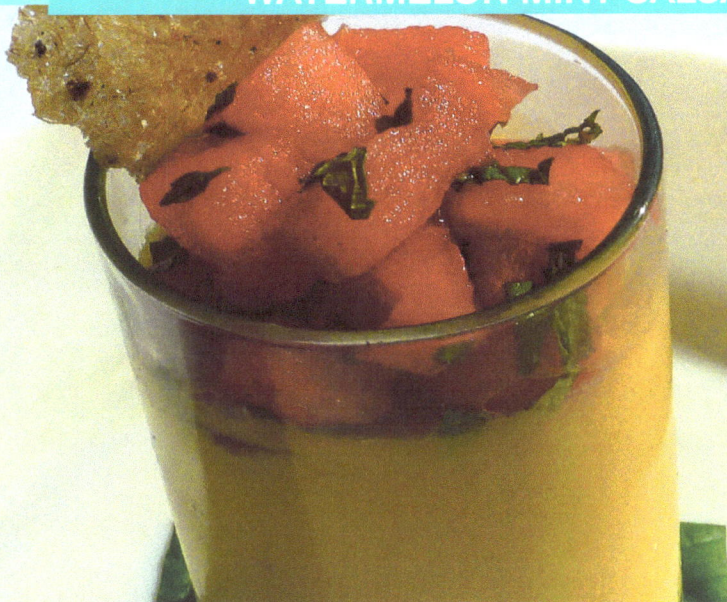

Preparation time: 15 mins

Cooking time: 20 mins

Total time: 35 mins

Yes you read right, oven baked coconut yoghurt! Once chilled and teamed with the minty watermelon salsa it truly is a taste and textural sensation!

Ingredients:

Serves 4

- 500ml (17 oz) coyo yoghurt
- 250gr (9 oz) watermelon (cut into cubes)
- Juice of ½ lime
- 250gr (9 oz) mango pulp
- 30gr (2 tbsp) chopped mint leaves

Method:

1. Pre-heat an oven to 150 degrees, (300 F).
2. Combine the yoghurt with the mango pulp and divide over serving glasses.
3. Place the glasses in an oven proof rimmed tray, add boiling water to the tray until the glasses are about 1/3 submerged.
4. Cover the glasses with aluminium foil and bake in the oven for 10 to 20 minutes, time depends on how cold the yoghurt is.
5. When you shake a glass gently and the yoghurt looks firm, it has set. Remove from the pan and cool for a few minutes.
6. Transfer the glasses to the fridge and allow cooling for a few hours, or overnight.
7. When ready to serve, combine the watermelon with the mint leaves and lime juice.
8. Divide over the yoghurt glasses and serve.

Nutritional values are manually calculated and based on the ingredients specified.
Nutritional value per serving: Calories: 245.4 Fat: 22.3g Saturated Fat: 0.1g. Sodium: 1.6mg. Sugar: 8.6g Carbohydrate 16.9g Protein: 3.4g Dietary fibre: 0.9g

SORBET

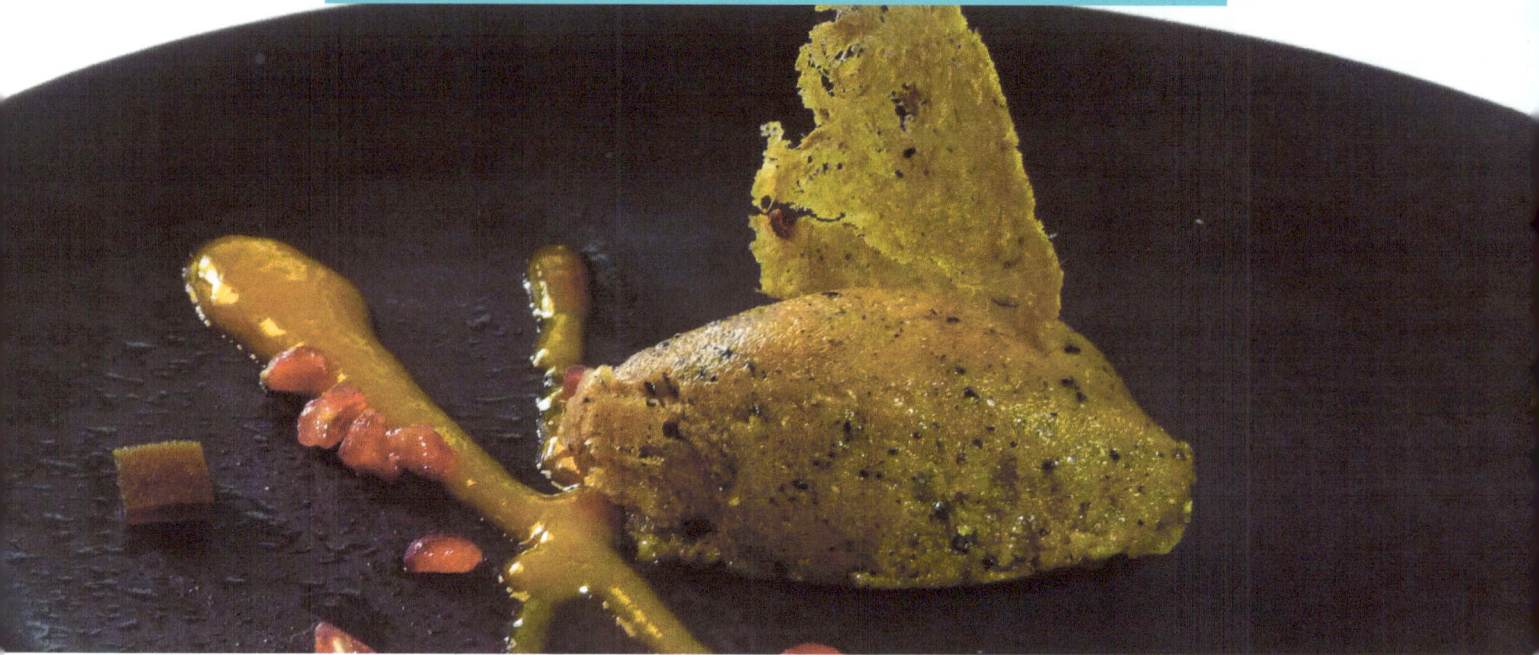

Preparation time:
15 mins

Total time:
15 mins plus
8 hrs Freezing time

Sorbet is a fantastic way to use up any fruit that is getting too soft. You can also add your sorbet to smoothies! If you have an ice cream maker put him on standby, if not, no worries, just scoop the mix around every hour or so. Just be sure to use a container with a lid to avoid ice crystal forming. Use any fruit you have, mixed fruit is also fine. How 'cool' is that!

Ingredients: Serves 4

- 900gr (2 pounds) of any fruit, I used kiwi fruit
- A few tbsp water

- 120gr (4 oz) coconut sugar

Method:

1. Bring the sugar with a few tablespoons of water to a soft boil, when the sugar has melted turn off the heat and allow cooling.
2. Clean the fruit you use and blend smooth.
3. Combine the fruit and sugar syrup and place in your ice cream maker. Follow the instructions that came with the machine.
4. If you don't have one, place the mix in a covered container and place in the freezer, mix every hour or so until frozen.
5. In case you have other things to do and you find a hard frozen block in the freezer when you check it later, just allow it to defrost a bit, break into small pieces and pulse smooth in a food processor.

Nutritional values are manually calculated and based on the ingredients specified.
Nutritional value per serving: Calories: 182.3 Fat: 1.0g Saturated Fat: 0.1g. Sodium: 11.3mg. Sugar: 12.0g Carbohydrate 45.5g Protein: 2.2g Dietary fibre: 4.7g

STEAMED BANANA COCONUT CAKES

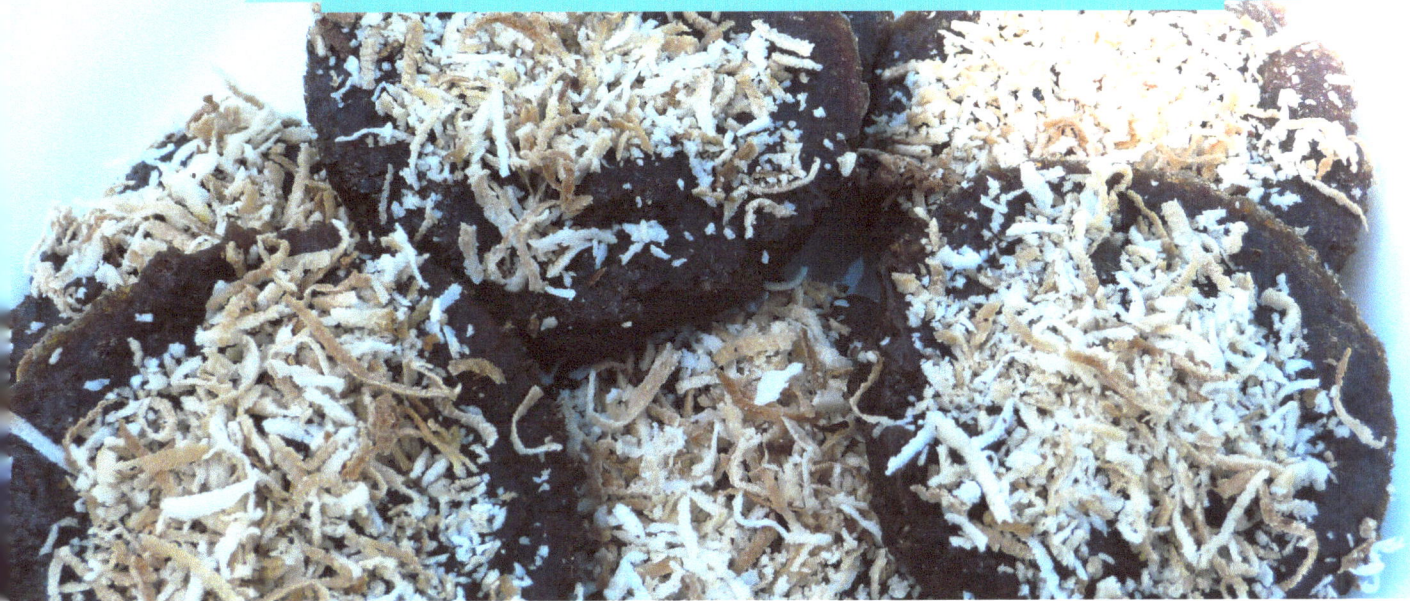

Preparation time: 15 mins	**Cooking time:** 15 mins	**Total time:** 30 mins

Baking without gluten and a raw protein like egg is not the easiest of tasks, yet with a little ingenuity there are some amazing dishes that can be created using AIP ingredients. Steaming sweetened coconut with agar-agar or tapioca flour is a common practice to make tea snacks in many Asian countries, and that is exactly what I did with these cakes. I just love the texture of these cakes, chewy and a little bit sticky.

Ingredients: Serves 4

- 60g (2 oz) banana flour
- 60g (2oz) grated coconut
- 50g (1 ¾ oz) tapioca flour

- 2 medium sized bananas
- 125g (½ cup) coconut cream
- Toasted coconut for garnish

Method:

1. Place all of the ingredients, except for the tapioca, in a food processor, you can use an up-right blender as well, but the blades may have some difficulty picking up the solids.
2. Blend into a smooth mixture and transfer into a mixing bowl.
3. Add the tapioca flour and whisk it firmly through, so it is well combined.
4. Spoon the mix in to small moulds about 1 ½ to 2 cm (¾ inch) thick. You can make one whole piece also and slice it later.
5. Place the cakes in a steamer, cover them with a lid and steam for 10 to 15 minutes. If you press on top with a finger and they are not sticky anymore they are done.
6. Allow cooling until you can handle the moulds, use a small knife or spatula to remove the cakes from the moulds.
7. Press them in the toasted coconut and serve.

Nutritional values are manually calculated and based on the ingredients specified.
Nutritional value per serving (one cake): Calories: 165.3 Fat: 4.6g Saturated Fat: 0.5g Sodium: 13.0mg. Sugar: 11.3g Carbohydrate 27.9g Protein: 1.0g Dietary fibre: 2.4g

TAPIOCA CREPES

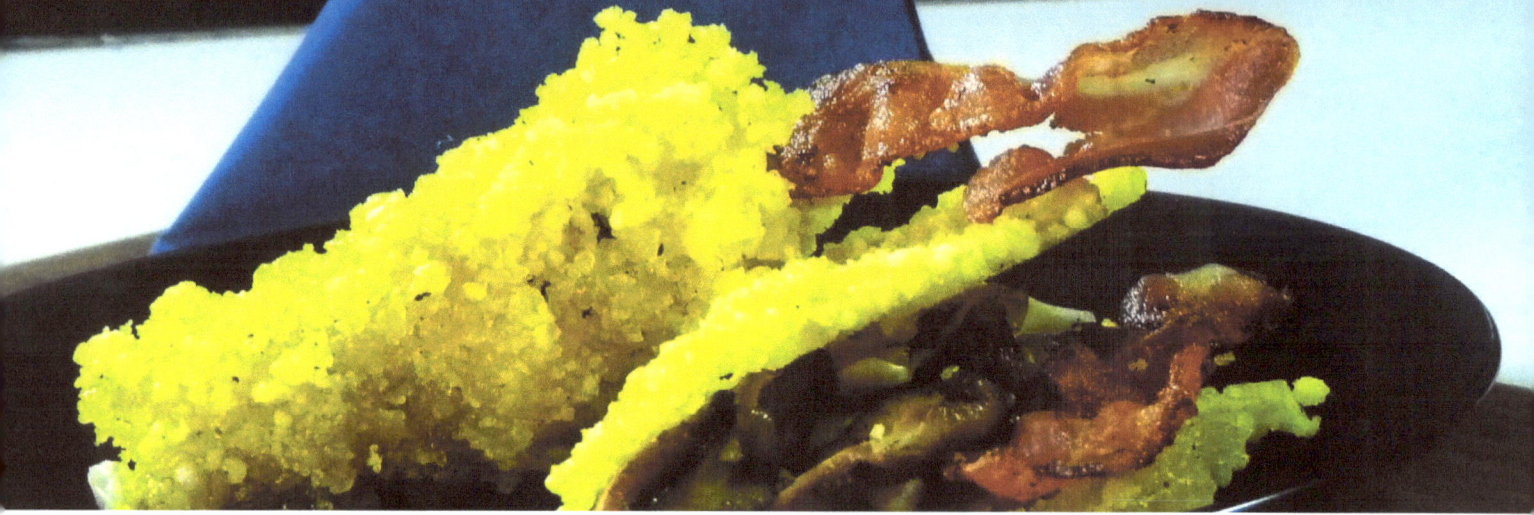

Preparation time: 10 mins

Cooking time: 10 mins

Total time: 20 mins

This is a very popular Brazilian street food that is served for breakfast, people just pick it up from a small road side stall and eat it while walking to work. Once you get the hang of the technique you will be making these all the time!! They come in a string of flavours, sweet and savoury, they cook very fast and you can roll them up like a burrito or just fold them like a tortilla. They are crispy, soft and delicious. When it comes to the filling and the size you can choose for yourself, I make mine with bacon, mushrooms and onion, but you can use a fruit filling such as berries!

Ingredients:

For 6 to 8 crepes
(depending on thickness and size)

- 250gr (1 cup) tapioca flour
- Little salt
- 6 to 8 tbsp water
- Oil for frying

Method:

1. Place the tapioca flour in a bowl with a little salt and sprinkle the water evenly over the flour.
2. Use your fingers to combine the flour with the water, the mix must remain fairly dry, the texture should somewhat be like a crumble.
3. Rub the crumble with the palms of your hands to make a very fine crumble. If you are not too sure about this you can rub the mix with your fingers through a sieve.
4. Grease a non-stick pan with a little oil and sprinkle some crumble evenly over the surface of the pan.
5. They cook quickly, about 20 to 30 seconds, just use a spatula to flip them over and crisp the other side.
6. Remove from the pan, add you're filling and fold or roll them up.
7. Best eaten hot and crisp.

Nutritional values are manually calculated and based on the ingredients specified.
Nutritional value per serving: Calories: 141.7 Fat: 1.8g Saturated Fat: 0.6g. Sodium: 66.9mg. Sugar: 0.0g Carbohydrate 35.8 g. Protein: 0.0 g. Dietary fibre: 0.7g

TARTE TATIN

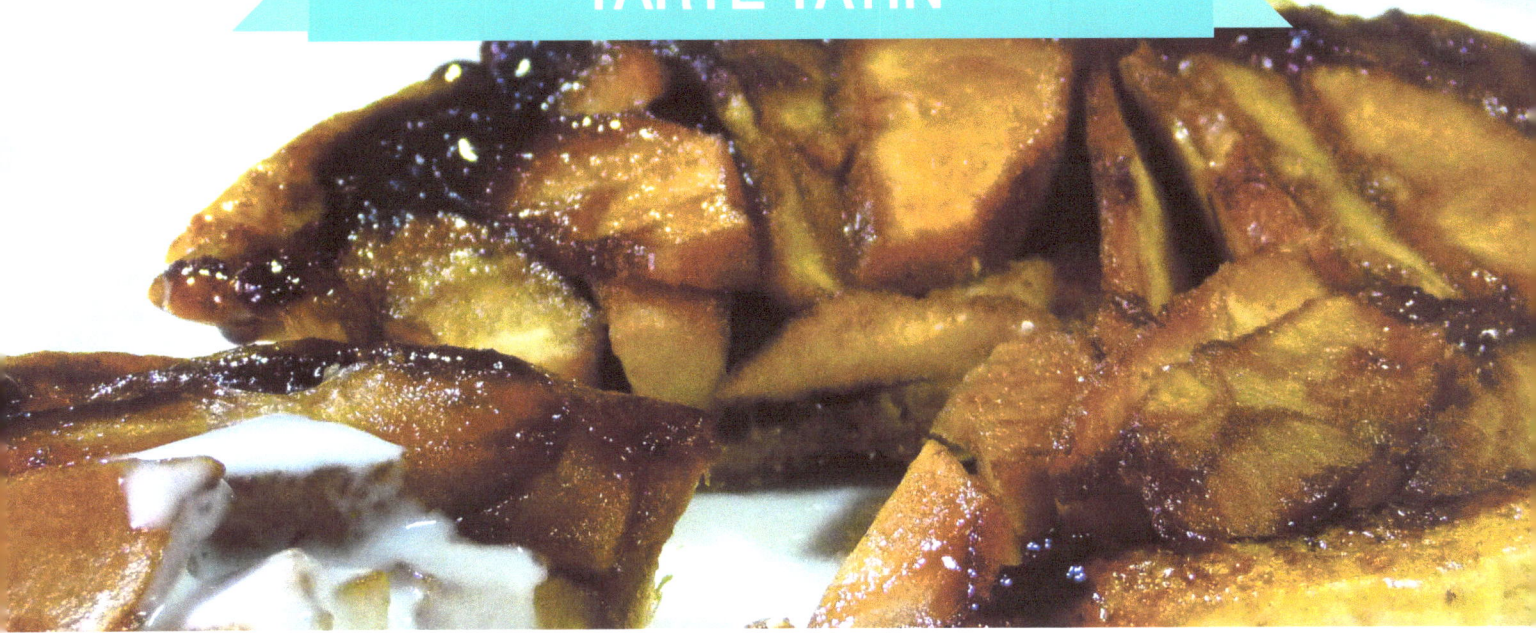

Preparation time: 25 mins

Cooking time: 25 mins

Total time: 50 mins

This is arguably the most famous tart that has ever been taken out of an oven! Being on an AIP protocol does not mean you should ever be deprived from having the pleasure of baking and eating one. This Tarte was one of the most popular desserts on offer at Vine. Even though it was a specified wait time of 30 mins to have these delectable creations made, diners were more than happy to wait! The twist on the pastry gives you the crispy flakiness you know and love in tarte tatin, without all those gut destroying ingredients! Please experiment with the fillings!

Ingredients:

For 6 to 8 crepes (depending on thickness and size)

- 150gr (5 oz) tapioca starch
- 200gr (¾ cup) fruit pulp (use a fibrous fruit, apple or pineapple works well)

- 2 large apples (cored, peeled and cut in splices)
- 60gr (2 tbsp) coconut sugar
- Juice and zest of ½ a lemon

Method:

1. Place your fruit in an up-right blender and pulse into a pulp. You may need to add a little water to allow the blender to pick-up the solids.
2. Transfer the pulp to a cheese cloth and squeeze some of the liquid out, you should have about 150gr (5 oz) of a fairly liquid pulp.
3. Add the tapioca starch and form into a dough. The ratio is about 1 to 1, depending on the liquidity of the pulp. You should have an easy to handle dough.
4. Grease a 20 cm (8 inch) baking pan and pre-heat an oven to 200 degrees (350 F).
5. Arrange the apple slices to the base of the baking pan, sprinkle the sugar, lemon juice and zest over the apples.
6. Roll the dough between two sheets of grease paper to the size of the baking pan.
7. Remove the top layer of paper and place the sheet with the dough up-side down on top of the apples. Remove the second sheet and press the dough along the sides of the apples. Bake for 20 to 25 minutes in the oven or until the crust has browned and is crisp.
8. Allow the tart to cool for a few minutes, then place a plate on top and turn the whole in one move up-side down.
9. Slice the tart in quarters and serve with a dollop of coconut cream.

Nutritional values are manually calculated and based on the ingredients specified.
Nutritional value per serving: Calories: 253.3 Fat: 1.5g Saturated Fat: 0.6g. Sodium: 29.2mg. Sugar: 22.1g Carbohydrate 61.3g Protein: 2.6g Dietary fibre: 2.6g

SMOOTHIES

BANANA, GINGER AND YOGHURT SMOOTHIE

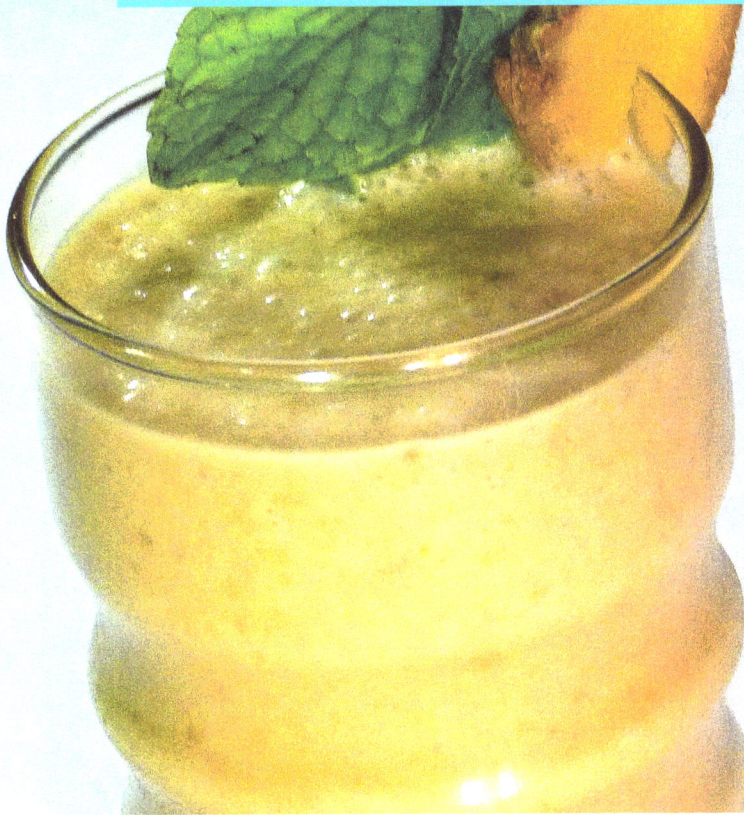

Preparation time: 15 mins

Cooking time: 01 mins

Total time: 16 mins

Smoothies are great as a breakfast booster to get you going for the day ahead. They also revitalize you after a workout and are just lovely refreshers when made with fresh fruit and yoghurt. For more gut healing and an extra protein hit, just add a couple of tablespoons of grass fed gelatin to your smoothies too.

Ingredients: Serves 4

- 4 medium sized bananas
- 60gr (2 tbsp) grated fresh young ginger

- 2 cups Coyo yoghurt

Method:

1. Place all of the ingredients in an up-right blender and blend smooth.

2. Serve in a tall glass.

Nutritional values are manually calculated and based on the ingredients specified.

Nutritional value per serving: Calories: 311.2 Fat: 23.5g Saturated Fat: 0.2g Sodium: 3.5mg. Sugar: 14.7g Carbohydrate 36.8g Protein: 4.4g Dietary fibre: 3.4g

GRAPE, WATERCRESS AND COCONUT SMOOTHIE

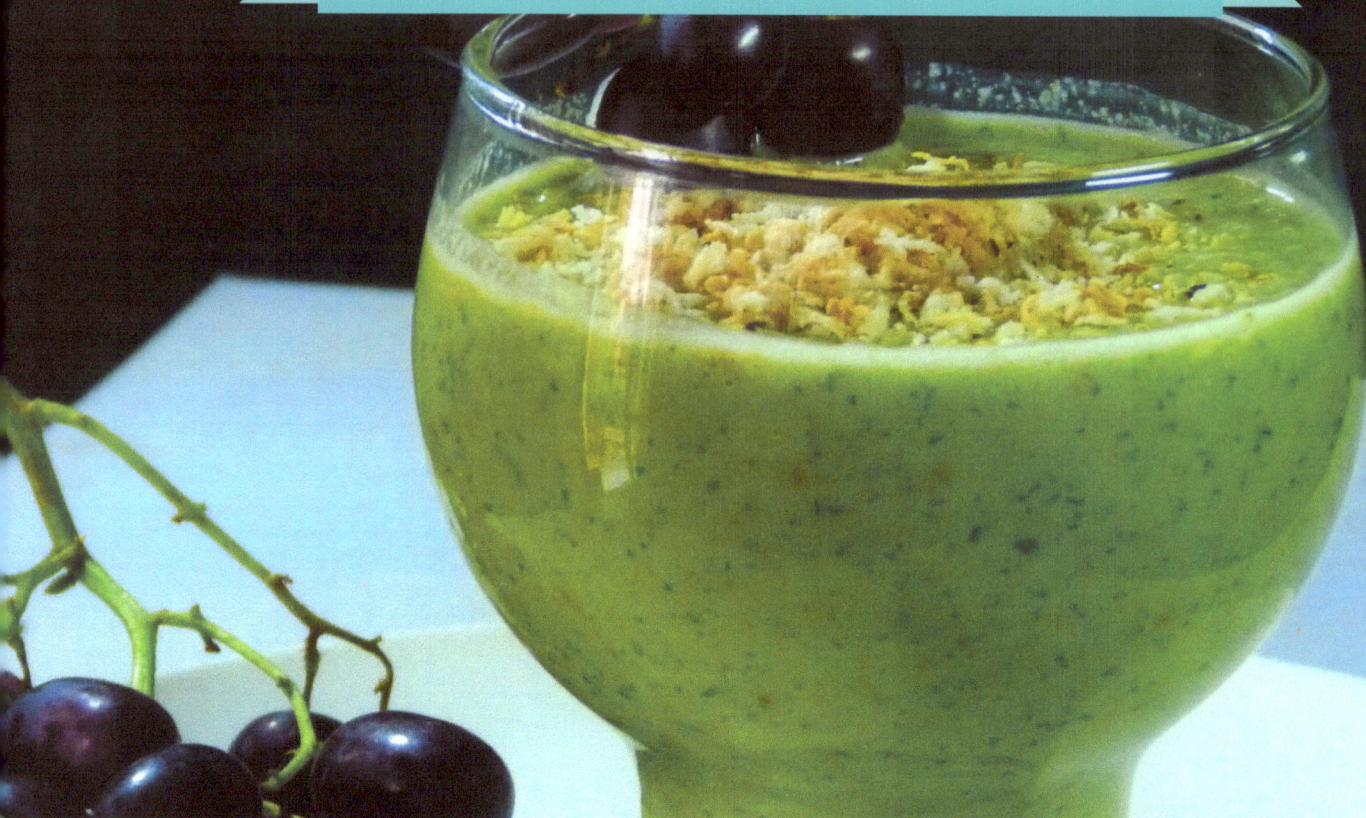

Preparation time: 05 mins

Cooking time: 05 mins

Total time: 10 mins

Quick and easy, this smoothie is packed with lots of nutrients and flavours. About the best way to kick start your day and it tastes delicious too.

Ingredients: Serves 4

- 500gr (2 cups) seed- less grapes
- 250 ml (1 cup) coconut milk
- 300gr (2 cups) watercress (stemmed)
- 90 ml (3 tbsp) maple syrup (optional)

Method:

1. When making smoothies always place the liquid first in your blender. This makes it easier for the blender blades to pick up all of the ingredients.
2. Place the cress and grapes in and blend until smooth and creamy.
3. You can adjust the consistency with some more coconut milk or water if necessary.
4. Serve the smoothie chilled.

Note: If you are in a hurry in the morning, make the smoothie the evening before and keep covered in your refrigerator.

Nutritional values are manually calculated and based on the ingredients specified.
Nutritional value per serving: Calories: 92.0 Fat: 1.4 g. Saturated Fat: 1.4 g.
Sodium: 17.3 mg. Sugar: 18.0 g Carbohydrate 20.3 g. Protein: 0.9 g. Dietary fibre: 0.5 g.

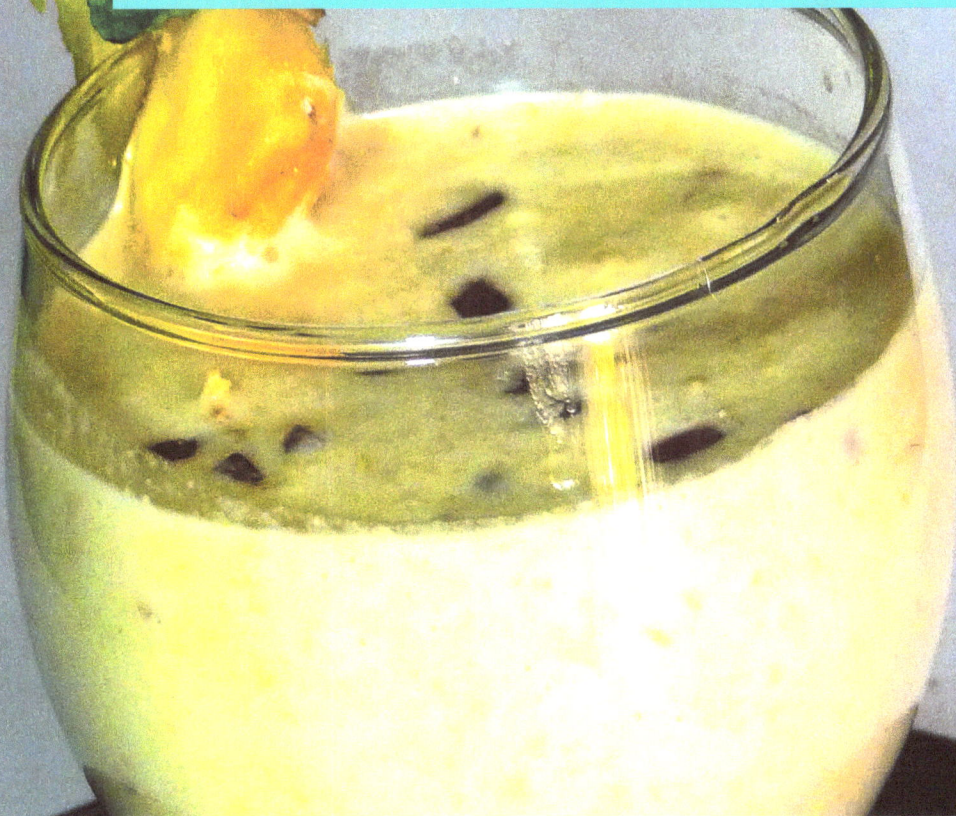

Preparation time: 15 mins

Cooking time: 01 mins

Total time: 16 mins

Pomegranate has very high amounts of antioxidants and is also thought to be very anti-inflammatory. Pomegranate is a fruit with little bullets of juice inside, every time you bite one you get a little explosion of juice in your mouth. This makes this smoothie an interesting and textural delight!

Ingredients:
For 2- 3 smoothies

- 25gr (1 cup) Coyo Yoghurt
- Kernels from one pomegranate
- 250gr (1 cup) coconut milk
- 250gr (1 cup) pineapple

Method:

1. Place the yoghurt, coconut milk, pineapple and half of the pomegranate in an up-right blender and blend smooth.

2. Divide the mix over glasses, add some pomegranate kernels to each glass and serve cold.

Nutritional values are manually calculated and based on the ingredients specified.
Nutritional value per serving: Calories: 101.2 Fat: 1.9g Saturated Fat: 1.7g Sodium: 14.7mg. Sugar: 10.3g Carbohydrate 20.9g Protein: 1.1g Dietary fibre: 2.4g

SWEET POTATO, COCONUT AND MANGO SMOOTHIE

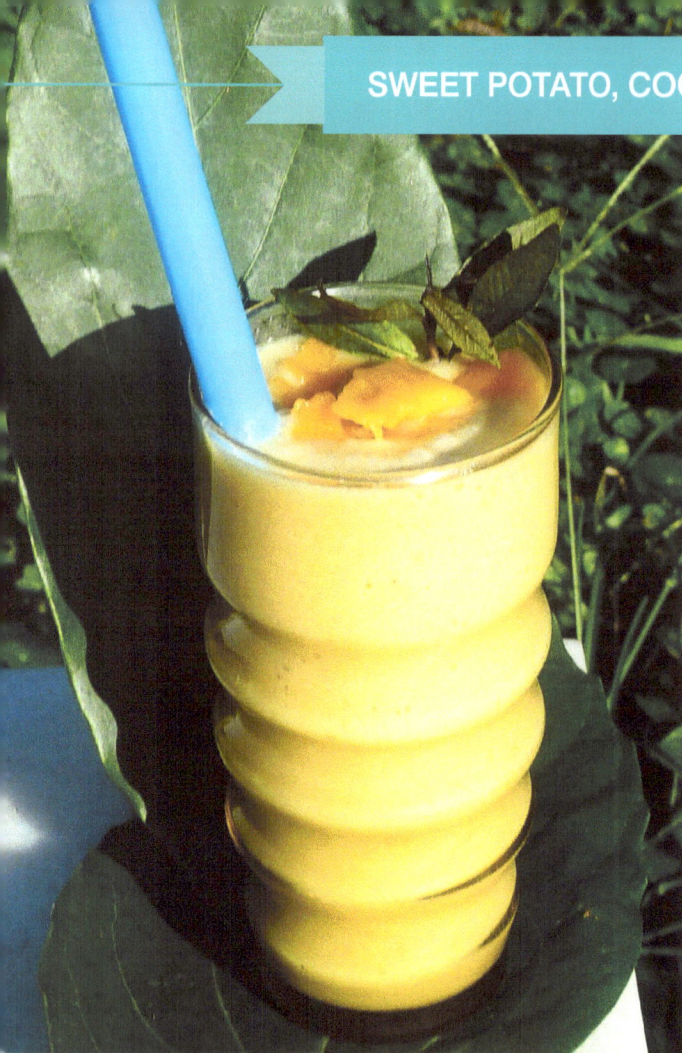

If you have never tried sweet potato in a smoothie then this a must try. Sweet potatoes are loaded with Beta-Carotene and Vitamin A; in fact 100g of sweet potato is enough to provide you with 90% of your recommended daily Vitamin A intake. The mango takes care of sweetness and taste and gives the smoothie a lovely colour.

Preparation time:
15 mins

Cooking time:
01 mins

Total time:
16 mins plus
chilling time

Ingredients: For 2- 3 smoothies

- 250g (1 cup) sweet potato (cut into cubes)
- 1 large mango (peeled and the flesh roughly cut)
- 3 ice cubes
- 250 ml (1 cup) coconut milk
- 125 ml (½ cup) water

Method:

1. Boil the sweet potato in water until soft, and then allow to chill in fridge.

2. Place all ingredients in an up-right blender and blend smooth.

3. Serve in a tall glass.

Nutritional values are manually calculated and based on the ingredients specified.
Nutritional value per serving: Calories: 101.2 Fat: 1.9g Saturated Fat: 1.7g Sodium: 14.7mg. Sugar: 10.3g Carbohydrate 20.9g Protein: 1.1g Dietary fibre: 2.4g

SPINACH AVOCADO AND APPLE SMOOTHIE

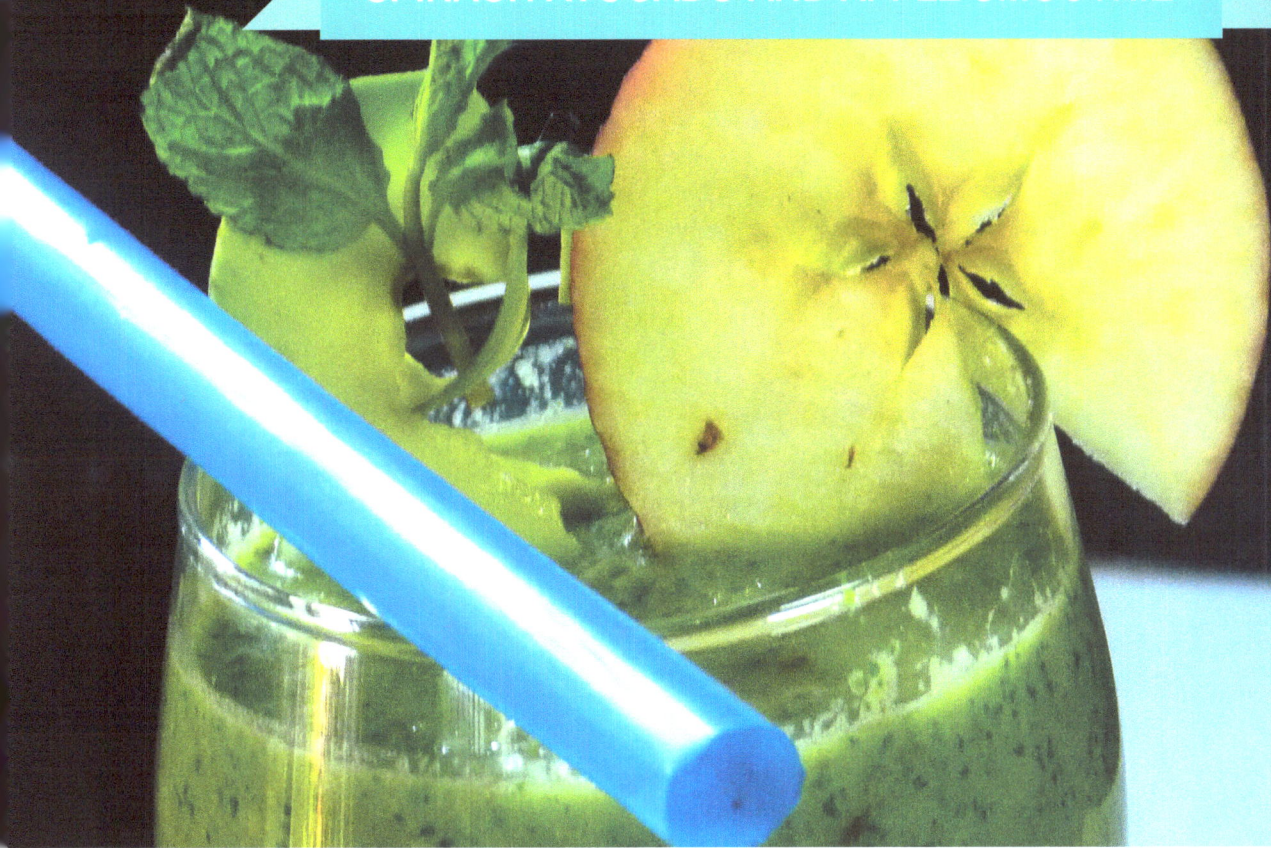

Preparation time: 05 mins

Cooking time: 05 mins

Total time: 10 mins

Juicy sweet apples spruce up this smoothie with avocado and vitamin rich spinach.

Ingredients:

- 750gr (3 cups) apples cored but skin-on (chopped)
- 125 ml (½ cup) apple juice
- 1 large avocado (skinned, de-seeded and cut in small pieces)
- 150gr (2 cups) baby spinach

Method:

1. Place the apple juice first in your blender, then top with the other ingredients and blend smooth.
2. You can adjust the consistency with some more apple juice or water if necessary.
3. Serve the smoothie chilled.

Nutritional values are manually calculated and based on the ingredients specified.
Nutritional value per serving: Calories: 152.2 Fat: 7.9 g. Saturated Fat: 1.5g. Sodium: 14.3 mg. Sugar: 10.5g. Carbohydrate 21.6 g. Protein: 2.3 g. Dietary fibre: 6.6 g.

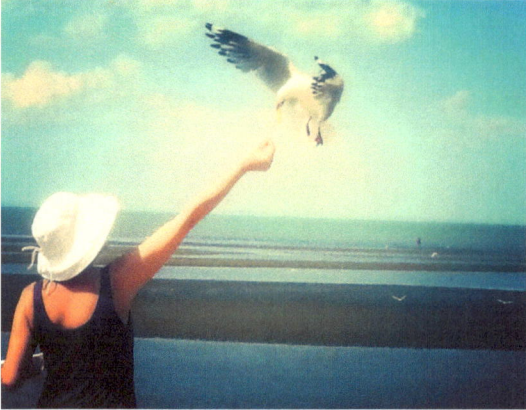

The inspiration for me to write this Australian AIP recipe book began after I adopted the AIP lifestyle. The trail blazers of the AIP community such as Mickey Tresscott, Eileen Laird and Dr. Sarah Ballantyne PhD had a plethora of amazing AIP recipes. The problem was they were, in many cases, quite difficult to adapt to our Australian seasonal produce and lifestyle. Many of the ingredients are simply not available in Australia. I have several friends with autoimmune and other chronic conditions, and they were amazed that my dishes had such unique flavour profiles and were so different to the AIP recipes available. I was constantly asked to share my recipes and even to show them how to prepare the dishes; at times even to cook for them! So with the overwhelming encouragement from my family and friends, the decision was made to write this book and share my AIP Australian culinary adventures.

My love affair with cooking first began when I was about 8 years old; I have fond memories of standing on my little wooden chair at the kitchen bench wearing a diving mask and snorkel, chopping onions!! I loved to experiment with different flavours and cooking techniques. I worked in one of the top fine dining a la carte restaurants in Brisbane for nearly 10 years, and much of my time there was helping in the kitchen and watching and learning from two of the best chefs in the City. The biggest thing I learned was that great food doesn't need to be complicated. You can make a world class dish with very simple ingredients. I want to share my expertise while bringing new dimensions to the AIP landscape. I want to show you that, even though you are embarking on a very restrictive elimination diet, it does not have to be bland or boring, even when you may be removing some of your absolute favourite flavours from your diet.

My Journey: In 1998 I was diagnosed with Hashimoto's disease and Chronic Anaemia, and I was more recently diagnosed with Addison's disease.

In 2014 due to major changes and stress, I endured one of the worst flares of my illness. I was so sick and tired I literally could not function. I had been seeing an integrated functional medicine doctor since my son was born in 2009. Pregnancy, childbirth and previous mismanagement in my treatment resulted in my being extremely unwell and barely functioning, while my list of symptoms seemed to be never ending.

I researched for thousands of hours, spent truck loads of money trying numerous supplements and treatments, while gradually gaining a sense of normality, or at least the closest thing to it. I simply struggled through to the best of my ability.

In 2014, after moving to the beautiful Sunshine Coast from Brisbane, the resulting stress of moving saw my body collapse from exhaustion. It started with a cold, then the flu, then infection after infection; I just couldn't seem to recover no matter how hard I tried. All my symptoms were so magnified; just doing the simplest task was overwhelming. After being so critically ill for nearly 7 months I was at the end of my tether. I have always relentlessly researched trying to find 'the key' to what I was missing to help me regain some enjoyment of my life. While researching, I stumbled upon Dr Terry Wahl's TED talk "Minding your Mitochondria" and this was my epiphany!!

I knew this was the answer for me. I read and studied everything I could about Paleo and Autoimmune Protocol Paleo (AIP). I figured in my haze of brain fog that I had nothing to change but the way I ate. With my chronic disease it was a better idea to go full AIP Paleo straight out of the gate! As there were no start up programs available at the time, the initial first four weeks was extremely difficult, what on earth was I supposed to eat???!!!!

Even though there are fantastic AIP warriors who have some great cookbooks, such as Mickey Trescott's Autoimmune Paleo Cookbook, I still found it quite difficult to find recipes that suited my tastes and our Australian way of life. Also our seasons are completely different and many ingredients are just simply not available here. I had to Google many ingredients to work out what they were or figure out a suitable substitute, which wasn't always possible. There were many days I was reduced to a puddle of tears of frustration but I persisted; giving up was never an option!

So once I got the hang of what flavours and ingredients I could use, instead of focusing on what I could not, I set about creating my own unique version of AIP. I am extremely proud of the recipes I have created. Many friends with Autoimmune Diseases and others that are simply health conscious love the dishes I have created, packed full of healing love and flavour. Get excited about going on a new healing journey with food as your medicine.

After my first 4 weeks on the Autoimmune Protocol and Paleo lifestyle I received the best blood work results in 17yrs! My doctor, who had been practicing functional medicine for 30 years was astounded! He said"I have never seen such an improvement in such a short time, from changing diet alone".

I am now over 18 months into living AIP and I have just received the amazing news that I am officially going into remission!! This news took me by surprise as I have been putting myself under a great deal of pressure and stress creating this book and the accompanying website. I had some routine blood work done and I received a call from the doctor's office to come and review the results. This made my heart sink as I have never received good news when being called in to get results. I had a 3 day wait to find out what was happening. Not unlike many autoimmune sufferers I struggle with anxiety, and it was a very long 3 days to say the least. When it was finally time for my appointment I was a bundle of nerves, then the totally unexpected happened. It was revealed that I have now the lowest antibody count I have ever had since my diagnosis. My doctor directly attributed my recovery and remission to strict adherence to the AIP, coupled with an integrated functional medicine approach. Finally, as I finish this labour of love, I have been given the greatest gift. All the frustration, tears, hard work, and above all unwavering perseverance has paid off, and it can happen for you too!!

I have provided support and information to many friends who have chronic disease who inspired me to help others. Seeing the results this lifestyle has had on me and my family (my husband has had a complete transformation; he has lost 28kgs/61lbs and reversed his type 2 diabetes and diverticulitis) and also my friends, I am totally convinced that everyone can benefit from the AIP Lifestyle.

After being on this AIP voyage for so long I decided to create www.Harmony-Hunter.com to help people find the missing key and provide an Australian perspective to help those with chronic disease, or those who simply want to live a vibrant healthy life.

Yours in Harmony and Good Health,

Natasha Horvath.

www.ingramcontent.com/pod-product-compliance
Lightning Source LLC
Chambersburg PA
CBHW061135030426
42334CB00003B/53